THRIVING

after

BREAST CANCER

THRIVING
after
BREAST CANCER

Essential Healing Exercises
for Body and Mind

by SHERRY LEBED DAVIS

with STEPHANIE GUNNING

BROADWAY BOOKS   NEW YORK

BROADWAY

The instructions and advice in this book are in no way intended as a substitute
for medical counseling. We advise the reader to consult with her doctor before beginning
any physical and/or mental rehabilitation program. The author and the publisher disclaim any
liability or loss, personal or otherwise, resulting from the procedures in this book.

THRIVING AFTER BREAST CANCER. Copyright © 2002 by Sherry Lebed Davis.
All rights reserved. No part of this book may be reproduced or transmitted in any form
or by any means, electronic or mechanical, including photocopying, recording, or by any
information storage and retrieval system, without written permission from the publisher.
For information, address Broadway Books, a division of Random House, Inc.,
1540 Broadway, New York, NY 10036.

Broadway Books titles may be purchased for business or promotional use
or for special sales. For information, please write to: Special Markets Department,
Random House, Inc., 1540 Broadway, New York, NY 10036.

PRINTED IN THE UNITED STATES OF AMERICA

BROADWAY BOOKS and its logo, a letter B bisected on the diagonal, are trademarks
of Broadway Books, a division of Random House, Inc.

Visit our website at www.broadwaybooks.com

First edition published 2002.

Designed by Lisa Sloane
Illustrated by David Ehlert
Photographs by Susan Picatti

Cataloging-in-Publication Data is on file with the Library of Congress.

ISBN 0-7679-0846-5

10 9 8 7 6 5 4 3 2 1

To my mother Rita Lebed:

Without her physical and emotional need for this program

and her desire to be a thriver, not merely a survivor,

this program could not have been developed.

To my brothers Dr. Marc Lebed and Dr. Joel Lebed,

who responded to my mother's needs and helped create

Focus on Healing: I love you both and thank you for the gift

of listening to your patients and to your sister.

CONTENTS

INTRODUCTION

Today I Am Alive and I'm Going to Thrive!

$\mathcal{M}$ore than twenty years ago I watched my mother, Rita Lebed, struggle to heal after a mastectomy. Once a professional ballroom dancer, she now had trouble lifting her arm and couldn't even perform simple everyday tasks or movements, such as hooking her bra. She was depressed and scared and felt as though she had lost control of her life. Despite the clinical success of her treatment, she was having trouble rejoicing that she had survived. It was difficult to witness such a vital person, someone for whom I cared deeply, become immobilized by pain and inflexibility.

On the phone one night, my two brothers and I came up with a plan to help our mother. Marc and Joel are both gynecological surgeons and I am a former professional dancer who at the time was running two dance studios. We decided to pool our talents and design an exercise program specifically for her needs. They would ensure it was medically sound; I would be the resource for the steps. Over the next few weeks, the program called Focus on Healing Through Movement and Dance for Breast Cancer Survivors (the Lebed Method) was born. We made it fun and safe by combining stretching with gentle movements from jazz dance and ballet. As my mother practiced the routines, her pain soon disappeared, her range of motion improved, and her dark moods lifted. We were elated by her success.

My mother's surgeon ran the breast clinic at Albert Einstein Medical Center in Philadelphia, Pennsylvania. He was so impressed with her progress that he asked us to start a program there. That year I began teaching a Focus on Healing class for breast cancer survivors at the hospital. I was proud that my family's creation could help so many women regain their strength, flexibility, and confidence. The response to Focus on Healing was overwhelmingly positive. In fact, it seemed to be the missing piece of the recovery puzzle.

At the time, very little research had been done on the importance of exercise to recovery, so a clinical research study was organized. Two hundred and sixteen participants between the ages of thirty and eighty-one were tracked through my program over a two-year period. When the physical therapy department completed the evaluation in 1984, they published their findings in the *National American Physical Therapy Journal* and the following year presented them at the National Physical Therapy Conference. The study proved that this program helps women recover from the physical side effects of breast surgery and treatment, such as tight scar tissue and stiff muscles. In addition, it improves posture and balance, reduces pain,

restores mobility, and increases vitality. It also gives breast cancer survivors a means to cope with their emotional stress and trauma.

Then in 1996, the teacher became the student. I had moved to Seattle in 1992 and recently married. When my doctor found a suspicious lump during a routine mammogram my first response was complete denial. Cancer was such a scary word that I was certain "It can't be me! This is a mistake." Then I did everything you are told not to do. Instead of going right into surgery, I went off on a weeklong vacation in the mountains with my husband, Jeff. I was experiencing a flood of contradictory emotions. Because I was convinced I was going to die, I actually persuaded him to buy a twelve-and-a-half-acre plot of land up there, where he could go to be happy "once I was gone," even though he didn't want it. It was located five hours from our home in a hot desert near some fruit orchards, and the bees were awful. During that week we cried a lot and held each other. I was trying to run away from cancer, but of course I had brought it with me. Then I came home and underwent the painful procedures of a lumpectomy with node dissection and radiation therapy. I was scared about the surgery and radiation, even though I knew they had to be done. I was hoping for the best outcome, yet I felt that my life had been forever altered.

I had thought I understood what a breast cancer patient goes through from being with my mother during her treatment and recovery and from teaching the Focus on Healing program to hundreds of survivors. I had listened to them talk about their lives and helped them as best I could. But now I gained new insight. The whole process was different from the other side. I felt sad and afraid, and I went through a period of intensely believing that I was going to die. For a while I lost my sense of femininity. There was too much happening, too fast, and on top of it all the side effects from my treatment overwhelmed me.

My surgical drain was in place for three weeks and it became all that I thought about. How do I take a shower? How do I get dressed? How do I sleep without disturbing it? Emptying the fluid revolted me. I didn't want to look at my wound, and when I did I cried. How ugly! My underarm was black and blue and my breast was bruised and deformed and there was a hole with a tube coming out of it. Thankfully, Jeff nursed me and offered a fresh pair of eyes. Each passing day he would tell me how much better it was looking.

I called my brothers in these early days, crying because I had lost my range of motion and was in pain. They reminded me, "You know what to do!" So I pulled my exercise regimen off the shelf and began practicing it religiously. The radiation therapy had exhausted me. I needed naps every day and my muscles and joints ached. But dancing and stretching made me feel as if I was going to live. It eased my pain, restored my flexibility, gave me energy, and helped me to release my emotions of loss and fear. Focus on Healing became my salvation. It helped me to look forward, not backward. I stopped dwelling on the worst that could have happened and began to focus on reality and what lay ahead. I had survived and I wanted to thrive. It was a cause for celebration, not despair.

Having experienced the benefits firsthand, I became passionate about sharing Focus on Healing with others. I contacted a hospital in my community and got the ball rolling again teaching classes to survivors three times a week. When I left Philadelphia six years earlier I had stopped teaching. Now I found that the program was even stronger because of what I learned during my own recovery. I made videotape and audiotape versions available in order to reach survivors everywhere. I phoned all the major cancer organizations to get them to approve and recommend my program to the women they served. I mailed these professionals the research article and sent them copies of the tapes. They were very interested. Soon survivors from all over the United States were contacting me and I was getting requests to train instructors.

In my classes I found that women were eager to share their stories. Only another survivor can truly understand the little things that gain such magnified importance when we cannot do them. These are the ordinary daily tasks that give us independence, such as being able to nurture and care for our children and spouses or holding down a job and bringing home income. Suffering from chronic pain and fatigue take a terrible toll. Surviving cancer is our first priority; the quality of the life that has been saved is second.

Most people are not aware of all the statistics that breast cancer survivors need to know:

◆ Up to 30 percent of the 2.5 million breast cancer survivors in the United States are likely to develop some symptoms of lymphedema at some point in their lives, according to the American Cancer Society.

◆ Women are often pushed into the advanced stages of menopause by their breast cancer treatments.

◆ Sixty percent of breast cancer survivors still feel depressed ten years after surgery.

◆ Many survivors lose their sense of balance as a result of surgery, which puts them at risk of falling and accidents, as well as neck and lower back problems.

◆ Too many survivors wear incorrectly fitted prosthetic breasts due to the poor training of sales personnel and being underinformed themselves. This causes discomfort, balancing problems, and makes the women feel unattractive.

There is a tremendous amount to learn once you have survived breast cancer. As one of my students told me not long ago, "Knowledge is strength." I wrote *Thriving After Breast Cancer* to give you knowledge that can make you stronger. Among other things, I hope it will answer the questions you have wanted to ask and never got the chance. Exercise is a major part of the solution to every single one of the issues listed above.

This book contains exercise routines, stories, and information that can help you heal physically and emotionally after breast cancer. All the photographs in this book are of women like you and me who are breast cancer survivors. Whether you are just out of surgery, in the middle of chemotherapy or radiation, or have been cancer-free for twenty years, there is something here for you. Whether you are young or old, have been active or inactive in the past, the movements here can help. I passed the five-year mark last year and I still find that if I don't do some gentle stretching and movement from the program at least three times a week, my pain comes back and my scar tissue gets tighter, so that I lose my full range of motion. Other survivors say the same.

Even years after surgery, the Focus on Healing program can help you:
◆ Regain and maintain your full range of motion
◆ Relieve the condition known as "frozen shoulder"

◆ Restore your physical and emotional balance
◆ Reduce your risk of developing lymphedema and relieve some of its swelling
◆ Raise your energy

Part One explains what you need to know before you begin the program, such as when it is medically safe to start exercising and which muscles the program targets. You will learn some important questions to ask your health-care provider. Other topics cover how to dress to work out, the importance of setting your own pace, how to prepare your environment, essential supplies, and musical selections. Perhaps most important, Part One includes a section called "Choosing the Right Workout" that guides you to and through the various exercise routines in later sections of the book. Finally, it also teaches you a critical sequence of exercises called the Basic Warm-up that you must do before any of the routines in the book, although it can also be used on its own and as preparation for everyday activities.

Part Two presents exercise routines targeted to the specific problems faced by survivors as we adjust to our new bodies, issues such as lack of flexibility, pain, loss of balance, and lymphedema. When you have recently undergone surgery and treatment, it's likely that you will benefit from starting with one of the routines in this section of the book. Then later, as your range of motion increases, your pain is reduced or alleviated, and your other problems also dissipate, you can begin doing the Ultimate Movements in Part Three. Part Two also contains workouts specially designed for women going through menopause and emotional upheaval, or who are seeking to celebrate their sense of femininity, as well as for those recovering from reconstructive surgery.

Part Three, "The Ultimate Movements," is just what the name implies, the ultimate complete exercise program for survivors who have achieved a full range of movement and are free of pain. It is divided into three sections: one targeted to the upper body, one targeted to the lower body, and one for building strength. You can perform these sections on their own or in combination. I recommend that you do each of them at least three times a week for the rest of your life for complete self-maintenance.

Every exercise program in Parts Two and Three is accompanied by a dance routine that is followed by a healing visualization or meditation. The dance steps are a unique feature of the Focus on Healing program. As a former professional dancer, I have always been deeply aware of the emotional and physical freedom and joy that come from dancing. It is an especially feminine form of expression to which the women in my classes genuinely respond. I love sharing my experience of dancing with other women. Throughout history many cultures have used dance as a sacred form of healing. You can use these dance routines to help you get in touch with and express your core feelings. Likewise, the guided visualizations and meditations are designed to facilitate your inward healing journey. I have included them as a way of honoring your commitment to your health and as an affirmation of your spirit and personal truth. Relaxation and positive imagery are proven techniques for healing and stress reduction.

This program is as much for active survivors as it is for recent postoperative survivors. Therefore, Part Four provides special warm-ups that can help you prepare for the demands of different sports. Participation in sports has many benefits. First, sports are fun. They can also teach us about the nature of resilience, persistence, teamwork, independence, and reaching for our goals.

And finally, because cancer recovery has many dimensions, Part Five addresses some other ways of taking care of yourself in addition to exercise. At the back of the book is a list of relevant resources and recommended reading.

Today I am a woman on a mission. I travel frequently to spread awareness of the importance of exercise for breast cancer survivors. The Focus on Healing program now runs in hospitals, cancer centers, fitness clubs, and community centers throughout the United States, Canada, and Korea. For information on becoming a certified instructor simply refer to the Resources section.

Above all, remember that you are not alone. You are part of a vast and growing sisterhood of survivors. Cancer recovery calls upon all our inner resources. It affects us on every level of our being. It is important to stay focused on being well, living well, and to keep moving. My dream is for this book to reignite your dance of life, and to help you stay strong, healthy, and invigorated for years to come.

No matter where I am going or what I am doing now, I always try to hold one idea in mind, especially when I feel challenged by obstacles. I hope you will also embrace it as you grow and heal and as you embark upon the program in these pages: Today I am alive and I'm going to thrive!

Sherry Lebed Davis

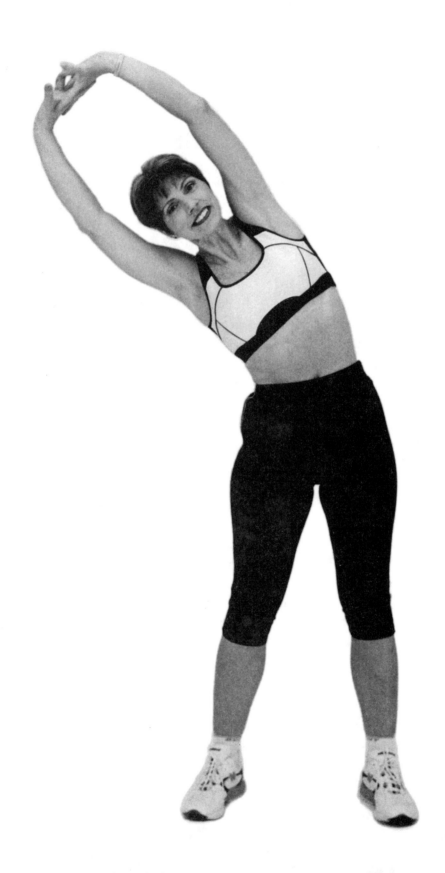

PART ONE

Getting Started

Fragile
I come for
Support
Caring
Fun
Laughter
Conversation
Healing

I leave with
Joy
Hope
Friends
Belonging
Strength

My body is
Stretched
Strengthened
Energized
Valued

My being is whole again
I am strong
I am ME

—BARBARA CUMMINGS-VERSAEVEL

BEFORE YOU BEGIN

$\mathcal{B}$y choosing this program you are honoring the needs of your body and making a commitment to the quality of your life. You have chosen to thrive. I salute you and I support you. I want you to have the safest and most pleasurable experience possible when you participate in the Focus on Healing exercise program.

As breast cancer survivors, we have unique needs and concerns. Some of these are physical and some are emotional. But none are a reason to avoid exercise. In fact, regular exercise can help with everything you feel and do. It can make you stronger and more flexible. It can relieve tension, elevate your mood, and give you a chance to celebrate and express your femininity. However, you must take your individual needs into consideration and exercise with care.

Your physiology has been changed by the type and extent of the surgery you have undergone. Lumpectomy, mastectomy, node dissection, and reconstruction all leave permanent imprints. Furthermore, your body may also be processing the radiation or chemotherapy that you received to treat your cancer. Perhaps it has been years since your surgery and you've been relatively inactive, or you are at risk for lymphedema—swelling that results from blockage in the lymphatic vessels—or have other health concerns. For these reasons it may be important to have a conversation with your doctor before you begin this or any other exercise program.

If you are a recent survivor, you may begin doing the Focus on Healing exercises as soon as your surgical drain is removed with the approval of your doctor. The surgical drain is a tube the size of a drinking straw that's inserted into your side a few inches below the armpit to siphon off excess lymphatic fluid. It has a bulb on the bottom. Sometimes you get two of them, the second being placed in the chest wall. A drain is kept in the body anywhere from three days to a week on average, until your body makes an adjustment.

Many surgeons have their patients begin doing simple arm movements during early recovery. These are extremely gentle and safe, as are the Focus on Healing exercises. Still, I recommend waiting until the drain is removed so that no unexpected complications occur at the site of your drain incision. It is a sensitive time and it is critical that you give your body the time to heal properly.

ABOUT THE PROGRAM Focus on Healing was designed under the supervision of two gyneco-logical surgeons, Marc Lebed, M.D., and Joel Lebed, D.O. Dr. Marc Lebed is currently the medical director of the program and ensures that it incorporates new advancements in medicine. The exercises are based on kinesiology (the science of movement), anatomy, and gentle ballet and jazz dance movements. Focus on Healing uses progressive patterns of passive and active arm movements to facilitate and improve your postoperative range of motion. It has been shown that these activities can also diminish your risk and incidence of lymphedema. In addition, lower-body exercises target muscles that enhance your posture and balance. The experience of doing the program is enjoyable and even sensual since it combines movement therapy with dance.

Focus on Healing works many important areas in your neck, shoulders, back, chest, torso, arms, hands, and fingers. The illustrations opposite identify the names of the muscles that are being used and receive benefits.

A CONVERSATION WITH YOUR DOCTOR You deserve special attention and expert advice from your physician. But what are the right questions to ask? Cheri Doll, a physical therapist from the Fox Chase Cancer Center in Philadelphia, Pennsylvania, suggests the following:

What kind of exercise should I do and what kind should I avoid? And when is the appropriate time for me to start exercising? Factors from your medical history that your physician will take into consideration include whether you are a recent or long-term survivor; whether you are currently undergoing chemo- or radiation therapy, your age, general health, and fitness; and whether you are a regular exerciser.

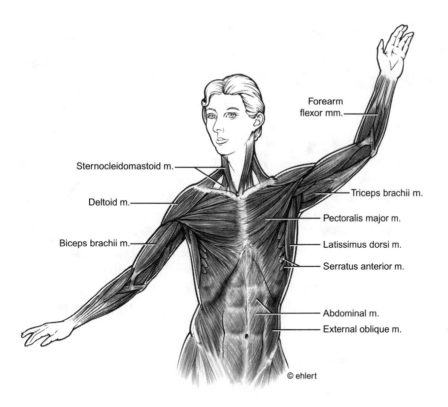

Forearm
flexor mm.

Sternocleidomastoid m.

Deltoid m.

Biceps brachii m.

Triceps brachii m.

Pectoralis major m.

Latissimus dorsi m.

Serratus anterior m.

Abdominal m.

External oblique m.

© ehlert

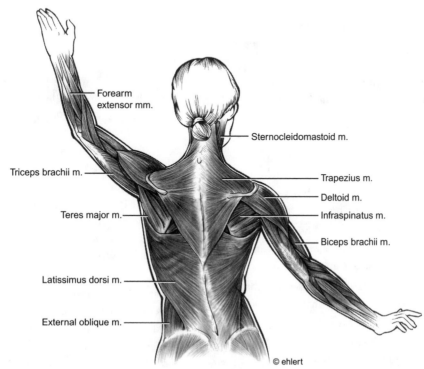

Forearm
extensor mm.

Sternocleidomastoid m.

Triceps brachii m.

Trapezius m.

Deltoid m.

Teres major m.

Infraspinatus m.

Biceps brachii m.

Latissimus dorsi m.

External oblique m.

© ehlert

EIGHTEEN STEPS TO PREVENT LYMPHEDEMA
ADAPTED FROM NATIONAL LYMPHEDEMA NETWORK

1. Absolutely do not ignore any slight increase of swelling in your arm, hand, fingers, neck, or chest wall. Consult your doctor immediately.

2. Never allow an injection, IV, or blood drawing in your affected or at-risk arm. Wear a lymphedema alert bracelet in case you are unconscious and cannot inform the people who are helping you. These are available from the National Lymphedema Network, (800) 541-3259.

3. Have your blood pressure checked in your unaffected arm, or on your thigh if you have bilateral lymphedema.

4. Keep your swollen or at-risk arm spotlessly clean. Use lotion after bathing. When drying your arm, be gentle but thorough. Make sure your arm is dry in any creases and between your fingers.

5. Avoid vigorous, repetitive movements against resistance with your affected arm (scrubbing, pushing, pulling).

6. Avoid heavy lifting with your affected arm. Never carry heavy handbags or bags with over-the-shoulder straps.

7. Do not wear tight jewelry or elastic bands around your affected arm or fingers.

8. Avoid extreme temperature changes when bathing (no saunas or hot tubs) or washing dishes. Keep your arm protected from the sun.

9. Avoid any type of trauma to your arm (bruising, cuts, sunburn or other burns, sports injuries, insect bites, cat scratches).

10. Wear gloves while doing housework, gardening, or any type of work that could result in minor injury.

11. When manicuring your nails, avoid cutting your cuticles. Inform your manicurist.

12. Do not overtire your at-risk arm. If it starts to ache, lie down and elevate it. Do not lift more than fifteen pounds.

13. When traveling by air, wear a compression sleeve if you have or are at-risk for lymphedema. Additional bandages may be required on a long flight. Increase your fluid intake while you are in the air.

14. If you have large breasts, wear light prosthetic breast forms. Heavy breast forms may put too much pressure on the lymph nodes above your collarbone. Soft pads may have to be worn under your bra strap. Wear a well-fitted bra that is not too tight and ideally does not contain an underwire. There are new bras available that have special wrappings around the underwire to protect you.

15. Use an electric razor to remove underarm hair. Maintain the razor properly, replacing heads as needed.

16. If you have been diagnosed with lymphedema, you should wear a well-fitted compression sleeve during all waking hours. At least every four to six months, see your lymphedema therapist for follow-up. If your sleeve becomes too loose, most likely your arm circumference has reduced or the sleeve is worn out.

17. *Warning*: If you notice a rash, blistering redness, or have an increase of temperature or fever, see your physician immediately. An inflammation or infection in your affected arm could be the beginning or worsening of lymphedema.

18. Maintain your ideal weight with a well-balanced, low-sodium, high-fiber diet. Avoid smoking and drinking alcoholic beverages. Your diet should contain protein that is easily digested, such as chicken, fish, or tofu.

How high can I lift my arm? And when? Your range of motion dictates the nature of the activities in which you can participate. Full range of motion means that you can lift your arm all the way up and slightly behind your ear while holding it close to your head. You can restore your flexibility through regular stretching, even when you have the extreme condition known as frozen shoulder. As I will repeat throughout the book, you should never do a movement that causes you pain. In a few pages I will help you assess what this means.

What is my weight restriction? How much weight can I lift with my surgical arm? And when? During recovery from surgery you lose strength and muscle tone and gain scar tissue. Radiation also tends to shorten the strands of the muscles. To exercise safely, you must know your limitations. You do not want to tear scar tissue while you are in the process of rebuilding your strength and flexibility.

What is my risk of lymphedema? Anyone who has had a lumpectomy, a simple mastectomy, a modified radical mastectomy, or axillary node dissection (the surgical removal of lymph nodes from the armpit), often combined with radiation, may be at risk for lymphedema. These treatments can reduce the functioning of your lymph nodes. Lymphedema can involve swelling of your breast/chest, arm, hand, and fingers and is caused by lymphatic fluid from your immune system pooling in these places. The swelling can result in discomfort. You can develop lymphedema at any time after surgery, from immediately to a couple of months afterward, or even twenty years or more down the road.

If you feel indications such as tingling and a tightness or fullness in your fingers, hands, arms, or chest, you should seek your doctor's attention and ask for a referral to see a lymphedema specialist. Lymphedema is incurable, painful, and sometimes leads to complications. It is a sign that your immune system has been compromised. Skin redness and the rapid onset of swelling, discomfort, and/or fever are signs of a possible infection, which must be evaluated as soon as possible. A certified lymphedema therapist can be a physical therapist, an occupational therapist, or a massage therapist who has trained in complete decongestive therapy. The National Lymphedema Network provides suggestions to the public on choosing a lymphedema therapist. You can call, write, or e-mail them to receive the information (see Resources).

The National Lymphedema Network has developed a comprehensive list of eighteen steps to prevent and control lymphedema. You should ask your doctor or a lymphedema therapist to review and discuss the list with you. Regular gentle exercise stimulates circulation and reroutes fluid to healthy pathways. It is therefore a key component of successful management.

A CONVERSATION WITH YOUR PHYSICAL THERAPIST OR OCCUPATIONAL THERAPIST Particularly when you're starting a new form of exercise, it is often advisable to seek the guidance of a physical or occupational therapist to help you overcome your challenges and monitor your progress. As you work through the Focus on Healing program, these trained professionals will know how to address your unique clinical needs. Your physician can give you a referral to a specialist.

An appropriate therapist must have experience working with other breast cancer survivors and understand your risk for lymphedema. Do not go to anyone without experience in the field. Before choosing a physical or occupational therapist review the Eighteen Steps to Prevent Lymphedema with the therapist and make sure your concerns are understood. Also ask the therapist to have a conversation with your surgeon.

SETTING YOUR OWN PACE No one can know your body as well as you, therefore you must set your own pace. If you feel pain, stop at once. Pain is an indicator that you are doing too much. Don't listen to the old adage "no pain, no gain." Focus on Healing is not based on this bad advice. When you are doing the exercises in this book I want you to concentrate on feeling better than you already do, not worse.

Likewise, if you feel out of breath, take a rest for a few moments or call it a day. Work only to the point where you become fatigued, and no further. Then stop and rest. Should you go past the point of fatigue, you may end up feeling exhausted at the end of the program. Whereas if you stop before you become fatigued, you will likely feel more energized. You don't have to prove to anyone that you are Wonder Woman. The goal here is to make steady, confident progress.

Please be patient and gentle with yourself. I promise you, your strength and endurance can and will increase over time. The human body is amazing. When it is called upon to work it musters resources to make the movements possible. Then it keeps a muscular memory of how it adapted to the challenge. So as long as you keep moving your body on a regular basis, it will continue to perform at the peak of its abilities.

Part of the program is aerobic, which means that you will find yourself breathing harder and that your heart rate has speeded up. It is a good idea to ask your doctor, a trained physical therapist, or another exercise professional to help you determine your target heart rate. This is the number of heartbeats per minute that you should reach but not exceed, and it depends on your age, weight, and level of fitness. It is different for everyone. You should take your pulse at intervals during the workouts to check how you are doing.

To check your heart rate, place two fingers flat against the inside of your wrist (your radial pulse point) or in the groove under your jaw (your carotid pulse point). You will know you're in the right spot if you feel a slight throbbing. Count the pulses for ten seconds, and then multiply the number by six. This is your actual heart rate.

When your actual heart rate is higher than your target heart rate, you should slow down or take a rest for a moment. When it is lower, you have the option of working harder should you choose to do so. Other indications that you are working too hard include shortness of breath long after you stop exercising or feeling undue fatigue and soreness long after exercise.

HOW TO DRESS FOR WORKING OUT There are no special outfits required to do this program. All you need are loose-fitting clothes and comfortable shoes without heels. Even doing the exercises barefoot is okay.

If you have a prosthetic breast form, you should wear it during the workouts. In order to develop a strong sense of balance, it is important to exercise the same way that you walk around in your daily life. If you have lymphedema, you must wear your sleeve to help keep your swelling under control.

PREPARING YOUR ENVIRONMENT You will need enough room to spread out your arms in every direction (plus a foot or two more for good measure). For most women this is approximately a six-foot-by-six-foot area. You should remove any obstacles within this space that you could accidentally hit or collide with while you are practicing your routines. Double check by turning in a slow circle.

You may also need to eliminate distractions. Turn off the telephone and shut the door to the room, if that helps. Ask your family to respect the time you have allotted for stretching and moving. This should be "you" time, so program a half hour into your schedule.

SUPPLIES Whenever you need a special item for an exercise, I clearly list it. Here are some of the items you may wish to have handy:

◆ **CHAIR:** Depending on which exercise routine you are doing, you may need a supporting chair for balance. Seated exercises are also included in some of the workouts. A kitchen-type chair without arms is preferred.

◆ **ELASTIC WORKOUT BAND:** See "Building Strength" (p. 176) for comprehensive details.

◆ **WATER:** It is beneficial to drink water frequently during and after your workouts.

◆ **TOWEL:** You may want this for your comfort when you perspire.

◆ **SOAP BUBBLES:** These are optional in Basics 1 (p. 15).

MUSICAL SELECTIONS Music is an important component of the Focus on Healing program. For one thing, music will elevate your spirits. But being able to follow a rhythm also supports the movements.

For the Basic Warm-up, which prepares you to do every routine in the Focus on Healing program, it would be helpful to pick something slow and flowing, such as classical music or ballads. For the rest of your workout, choose something with a faster tempo. Music that has four main beats works best. Let it be music that makes you want to dance—whatever gets your toes and fingers tapping, head bobbing, or hips swinging. Varying your musical selections from time to time will help keep the program fresh.

The survivors and instructors from Focus on Healing classes throughout North America have given me a list of their favorite CDs and performers. Often they prepare their own song mixes for the program on a cassette tape or CD. These suggestions may guide you in your own selections.

SLOW MUSIC
◆ *The Best of Doo Wop* (Rhino)
◆ Michael Bolton, *Love Songs*
◆ Sarah Brightman, *Time to Say Goodbye*
◆ *Down in the Delta* (movie soundtrack)
◆ *Fall* (Telarc)
◆ Kenny G, *Classics in the Key of G*
◆ Herbie Hancock, *Gershwin's World*

- ◆ Frank Sinatra, *Swinging Around the World*
- ◆ *Spring* (Telarc)
- ◆ Barbra Streisand, *Barbra Back to Broadway*
- ◆ *Summer* (Telarc)
- ◆ Vangelis, *Escapes*
- ◆ *Where the Heart Is* (movie soundtrack)
- ◆ *Winter* (Telarc)
- ◆ Zamfir, *Intemporal*

MUSIC ON THE WEB:

Music is now available over the Internet. Visit these websites.

- ◆ www.dynamixmusic.com
- ◆ www.powermusic.com
- ◆ www.musicflex.com

FAST MUSIC

- ◆ Abba, *More Abba Gold*
- ◆ Lou Bega, *Little Bit of Mambo*
- ◆ Ray Charles, *Visionary Soul*
- ◆ *The Conga Kings* (Chesky Jazz)
- ◆ *Dance with Me* (movie soundtrack)
- ◆ Gloria Estefan, *Gloria*
- ◆ Fleetwood Mac, *Greatest Hits*
- ◆ Aretha Franklin, *Love Songs*
- ◆ "I Feel Pretty" (*West Side Story* cast recording)
- ◆ Tom Jones, *The Complete Tom Jones*
- ◆ Jennifer Lopez, *On the 6*
- ◆ Ricki Martin, *Livin La Vida Loca*
- ◆ Ricki Martin, *Sound Loaded*
- ◆ Mary Mary, *Thankful*
- ◆ Dolly Parton, *Nine to Five and Odd Jobs*
- ◆ Santana, *Supernatural*

- ◆ *Saturday Night Fever* (movie soundtrack)
- ◆ Donna Summers, *Alive and More*
- ◆ *Swing* (cast recording)
- ◆ Manhattan Transfer, *The Swing*
- ◆ *VH-1 Divas Live '99* (BMG/Arista)

CHOOSING THE RIGHT WORKOUT Now you are ready to begin the Focus on Healing exercises. Start with the Basic Warm-up in the next section. The Basic Warm-up is the first thing you should do every time you exercise, whether you are still in treatment or a long-term survivor. It gently establishes your breathing pattern and increases your circulation.

Then choose a full-length workout program that fits your special needs from Part Two, "Adjusting to the Needs of Your New Body," or do the full-length program from Part Three, "The Ultimate Movements." It's a good idea to stick with the same program for as many days or weeks as it takes to perform it successfully. Above each of the programs there is detailed information to help you determine when that program is suitable for you and what you need to keep in mind as you do it. Here is some additional guidance:

FOCUS ON HEALING CLASS CD

We created a CD for Focus on Healing classes called *Rhythmic Accompaniments to Focus on Healing Through Movement and Dance* by Randy Gloss, which may be ordered toll free through Focus on Healing (see Resources).

"RESTORING FLEXIBILITY": Loss of range of motion is the most common problem faced by breast cancer survivors. It can lead to other problems, so it's a good idea to address it head-on. Postoperative survivors often find they've lost mobility from the procedure and/or other treatments. Long-term survivors may never have regained their full range of motion or, for other reasons, such as scar tissue and pain, have become more inflexible over time. Use this program to increase your mobility whenever you feel tight or if you have a frozen shoulder, unless you have just had reconstructive surgery (see "After Reconstruction" below).

"MOVING THROUGH PAIN": Pain can be a tremendous problem soon after surgery and during radiation therapy and chemotherapy. But it can also be a problem for long-term survivors, especially those who have been inactive. Pain is a subjective issue. Use this program if you feel that pain is your greatest obstacle to movement, otherwise begin with "Restoring Flexibility" (p. 29).

"COMBATING FATIGUE": Women undergoing chemo- and radiation therapy often feel very tired. This program is designed to boost your energy, and all of the exercises in it can be done while seated. Use it first, before doing other programs, if exhaustion is your greatest challenge.

"EMOTIONAL RECOVERY": For women who are feeling depressed or angry, it is just as important to unload emotional baggage as it is to recover flexibility, stamina, and strength. Use this pro-gram when your emotions are getting in the way of living your life to the fullest. If you have recently undergone surgery or are still undergoing radiation or chemotherapy, you may alternate this program with the programs for "Restoring Flexibility" or "Moving Through Pain" (p. 49). If you are a long-term survivor and have progressed far enough, you may alternate it with the "Ultimate Movements" (p. 154). For example, you could do "Emotional Recovery" (p. 75) on Monday and Thursday and "Restoring Flexibility" on Wednesday and Saturday.

"LIVING WITH LYMPHEDEMA": If you have been diagnosed with lymphedema, use this program until most of the swelling and pain subsides. Then you can move on to other programs, such as "Restoring Flexibility."

"DEVELOPING BALANCE": Breast surgery changes the body's weight distribution. This can be disorienting and lead to discomfort when the body tries to compensate for the change. Use this program if you notice that you are experiencing neck or back problems, your shoulders are uneven, or you feel wobbly or dizzy when you are walking or standing still. Getting your balance under control doesn't take very long once you discover your new center of gravity. Then you can go on to other programs.

"MENOPAUSE": One of the most unwelcome side effects of breast cancer treatment and cancer prevention drugs is early menopause, including the same range of symptoms as natural menopause, such as hot flashes, mood swings, and night sweats. Use this program if your menopausal symptoms are out of control and getting in the way of your daily activities. Feel free to switch off doing this program with another one like "Restoring Flexibility" or the "Ultimate Movements" if you have progressed that far.

"EXPLORING YOUR FEMININITY": Breast cancer survivors too often feel as though their femininity has been taken from them. Use this program when you want to boost your sexual energy or libido, or simply to celebrate the joy of being a woman. As with the "Emotional Recovery" and "Menopause" programs, you may alternate this program with those that target other issues.

"AFTER RECONSTRUCTION": Reconstructive surgery is sometimes done at the same time as the original cancer surgery and sometimes it is done later. This kind of surgery can be quite extreme, so survivors need to begin exercising very cautiously and gently afterward. Use this program for at least six months after your reconstruction.

You should only move on to other programs with the permission of your doctor.

"THE ULTIMATE MOVEMENTS": Once you have achieved full range of motion and are pain-free, you can begin doing this full-length program—unless you have lymphedema or trouble balancing. Feel free to mix and match the exercises with dance routines from the other workout sections for variety. They are all appropriate for you. Have fun!

Women who are currently in postsurgical treatment should begin one of these exercise routines after their surgical drains have been removed. However, if you are in the midst of a course of chemo- or radiation therapy, consider doing only half a workout program so as to conserve and boost your energy. Follow the guidelines above to select an appropriate program, and remember always to prepare for your workout with the Basic Warm-up.

THE BASIC WARM-UP

"There are things I can do today that I couldn't before Focus on Healing, such as reaching the second and third shelves in my cupboards and hooking my bra in the back. Now, before I do vacuuming or gardening, I do the warm-up exercises, and the next day I'm not hurting."

—Debbie, thirty-eight

The Basic Warm-up is a short warm-up routine to use before doing any of the movement programs in this book, before playing sports, or before any other physical activity. It is also a good idea to do the Basic Warm-up before everyday tasks like housework, gardening, and child care. A simple warm-up prepares your body to move and helps prevent injury.

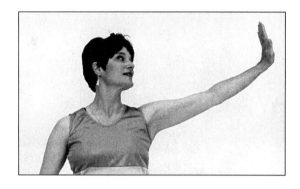

FLEXING YOUR WRIST In many exercises I ask you to keep your wrist flexed. The purpose is to stretch the tendon that runs along the inside of your arm from the wrist to the armpit. This is particularly important for those who have had node dissection and radiation therapy, since from time to time scar tissue can spontaneously develop along this tendon. This kind of scar tissue forms a long, rigid line that feels like a kite string. If you do your exercises with a flexed wrist, the stiff tissue breaks up and the line should disappear.

GOOD POSTURE It is important to maintain good posture as you do the exercises. This is critical for breast cancer survivors because surgery can change the distribution of weight between the right and left sides, and also because we may be physically compensating in several ways for the pain and inflexibility we often feel on the surgical side. Over time these awkward holding patterns can get locked into our muscles and put stress on the neck and the spine.

Good posture means that when you are standing or seated your spine is straight. Your head and shoulders are level, not tilted. Your shoulders should be pressed down evenly and held back slightly. Imagine that your shoulder blades are pinching together a bit so that your body doesn't

round forward and your chest remains open. You should also suck in your stomach slightly, as if you're trying to zip up a tight pair of jeans. But don't forget to breathe!

DOING THE BASIC WARM-UP The first six Basics are designed to boost your circulation and deepen your breathing. They increase blood flow and begin to open the lymphatic system so your fluids can drain properly and cleanse your body. The next three Basics are designed to gently stretch your scar tissue, helping you maintain and regain your range of motion. You may perform the Basic Warm-up seated or standing, depending on the special needs of your own body.

Please remember to go easy on yourself when you are recovering from recent surgery. Pay attention to how you're feeling today. Are you sore? Tight? Tired? Rest assured, over time you will become more flexible, your energy levels will improve, and your pain will gradually abate.

MUSICAL SUGGESTION: I recommend that you perform the Basic Warm-up slowly and gracefully to soothing classical music or your favorite ballads.

THE BASIC WARM-UP
◆ Breathing
◆ Neck Stretch
◆ Shoulder Rolls
◆ Shoulder Shrugs
◆ Chest Contractions and Expansions
◆ Side Isolation Stretch
◆ Arm and Torso Lengthening
◆ Large Arm Circles to the Front
◆ Large Arm Circles to the Side

BREATHING

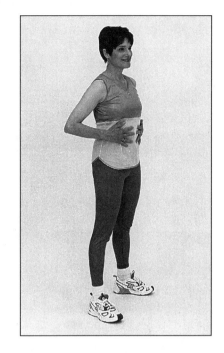

Before you begin exercising, it's important to open up your chest and lungs. Why? Your muscles need oxygen to perform well. Breathing also boosts the immune system, which is particularly beneficial if you've recently been under anesthesia during surgery, taking chemotherapy, or getting radiation. Deep breaths can both energize and relax you.

This short exercise sets the breathing pattern for your entire workout. During the rest of your movement session, when I remind you to breathe, this is what I mean.

In our society women are often trained to hold their stomachs in at all costs. Unlike the other exercises I'll give you, in this exercise you need to allow your stomach muscles to relax and be open.

WHAT YOU NEED FOR THIS EXERCISE: Soap bubbles are optional.

STARTING POSITION: Stand with your feet hip-width apart, or sit in a chair with your feet flat on the floor. Take a moment to check your posture. Is your spine straight? You should not be slouched forward. Are your shoulders pressed down? Are they even? Your head should be level—tipped neither forward nor back. It can help to pick a spot on the wall where you can place your sight line. Rest your hands on the lower part of your rib cage at first to feel the movement of your belly.

STEP 1: Inhale through your nose on a slow count of three. Feel your stomach expand outward. Then exhale through your mouth, also on a slow count of three. As you release air, pull your stomach muscles tightly inward. Repeat four times.

As you get more practice, see if you can increase the length of your inhalation and exhalation to five, six, or more counts. For fun, try using soap bubbles to help you see what's happening with your breath. A fifty-six-year-old survivor in my class likes to sit on her deck outside and blow bubbles when she's upset or needs a quiet moment. The stream of her breath goes on for eight counts now. She says the bubbles make her feel like a happy kid.

POINTERS:

◆ Your inhalation and exhalation should form one continuous cycle and be of equal duration. It's not necessary to hold either the in-breath or the out-breath.

◆ It's normal for some people to get a little light-headed. It only means that you're getting more oxygen than you're used to— and that's a good thing. Feel free to stop and rest. If you're dizzy, you can put your head between your knees. When you practice breathing every day you'll find you soon adapt to it.

NECK STRETCH

Your emotions and body are inextricably linked. Particularly when you feel threatened or are under stress, you tend to collapse your posture inward or tense up the muscles in your neck and shoulders. This exercise helps release any tension you may be holding in these spots.

STARTING POSITION: Stand with your feet hip-width apart, or sit with your feet flat on the floor. Your hands can hang down or rest on your hips, depending on which position you find most comfortable.

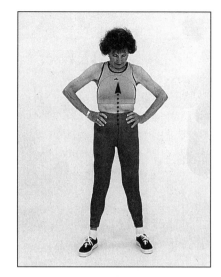

STEP 1: Slowly tilt your head forward so that your chin touches your chest. Hold it in this position and breathe. Then raise your head to the starting position.

STEP 2: Gently tilt your head toward your right shoulder. Hold it in this position and breathe. Return to the starting position. Then gently tilt your head to the left. Hold it in this position and breathe. Return to the starting position.

STEP 3: Slowly turn your head to the right, as if you're checking for cars when crossing the street. Hold and breathe. Return to center. Finally, turn your head to the left. Hold and breathe. Return to center.

Repeat.

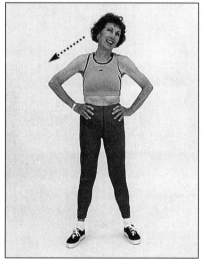

POINTERS:

◆ Maintain good posture. Keep your shoulders still and let your head do the work.

◆ Please don't strain. If you can't get your head all the way forward, for instance, work toward this position as a longer-term goal.

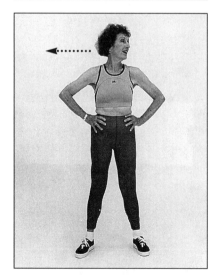

SHOULDER ROLLS

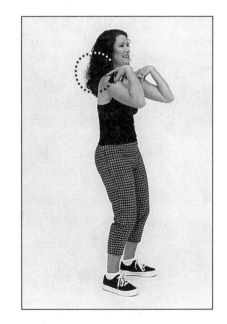

Besides being generally relaxing, Shoulder Rolls help your chest muscles to expand. Stretching out the scar tissue in this way begins to loosen up your shoulders.

STARTING POSITION: Stand or sit with your feet hip-width apart. Bend your arms and place your fingertips on your shoulders, elbows pointing to the front, while maintaining good posture.

COUNTS: Every Shoulder Roll takes four counts.

STEP 1: Circle your elbows up and out to the side, then back and down, allowing your shoulders to roll with them. Do four rolls. Now, do four rolls circling in the opposite direction.

POINTERS:

◆ You can also do Shoulder Rolls without lifting your arms, by just letting them hang at your sides instead. Just make it a point to keep your chest lifted.

◆ Remember to keep breathing.

SHOULDER SHRUGS

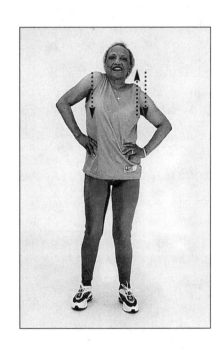

I sometimes get tied up in knots trying to manage all the details of my daily routine. And like many of you, I often feel as though I'm literally carrying the weight of the world on my shoulders. Shoulder Shrugs target this problem area. They are also wonderful for posture.

STARTING POSITION: Stand with your feet hip-width apart. Rest your hands lightly on your hips. Your shoulders must remain level.

COUNTS: Every shrug takes four counts.

STEP 1: Slowly lift your right shoulder up to meet your right ear—without tipping your head. Release it slowly and gently press it down. Repeat four times.

STEP 2: Next, slowly lift your left shoulder up to meet your left ear. Release it slowly and gently press it down. Repeat four times.

STEP 3: Alternate shrugging your right and left shoulders four times.

POINTERS:

◆ If you choose to do your warm-up to fast music, it's advisable to perform this series of movements at half speed rather than on the beat. It should not be an aggressive movement.

◆ Concentrate on isolating your shoulders. In order to reap the greatest benefits, your resting shoulder should remain level and your head upright.

CHEST CONTRACTIONS AND EXPANSIONS

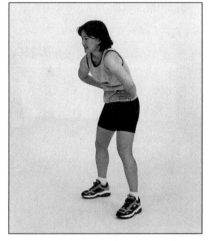

The Chest Contractions and Expansions are complementary movements for the neck, shoulders, chest, and back. You are opening up the lymphatic system throughout the upper torso during this exercise. You are also waking up the spine, which should enhance your flexibility.

STARTING POSITION: Stand with your feet hip-width apart and your knees slightly bent. Or sit forward on your chair in a firmly grounded position. You'll be moving your body above the waistline, so place your hands on your hips to help stabilize your base. Your shoulders should be down and even.

COUNTS: Every movement takes two counts.

STEP 1: Pull in your stomach muscles, as if you have been punched in the stomach, in slow motion. Let your shoulders hunch over. Focus on your back expanding. Then slowly return to the starting position.

STEP 2: Next, expand your chest forward and upward, as if you are very proud of yourself. Press your shoulders back. Slowly return to the starting position.

Repeat four times.

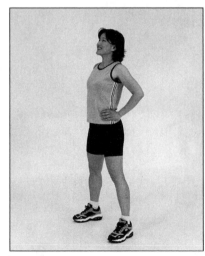

POINTERS:

◆ Allow your head to follow your shoulders naturally as you move them forward and backward. Look down and look up.

◆ You can tuck your butt and hips under you a bit if you feel that it gives you a fuller stretch.

SIDE ISOLATION STRETCH

Here you will be making the same kind of movements as in the Chest Contractions and Expansions, except you will be going to the right and left. The purpose is to get a good stretch along the sides of your rib cage and above your hips.

STARTING POSITION: Stand with your feet about three feet apart. Your toes are pointed out. Keep your resting arm on your hip. Or you may sit with your feet hip-width apart.

COUNTS: Every movement takes two counts.

STEP 1: Bend your right knee slightly and shift your rib cage to the right. As you move, raise your right arm to shoulder height and extend it out to the side until you feel a pull in that direction. It is as though you are trying to grab something that's a little out of reach. Hold for two counts. Then return to center and lower your arm.

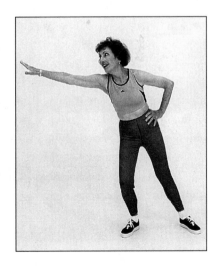

STEP 2: Repeat the stretch on the other side, bending your left knee and extending your left arm out to the side.

Do two sets.

POINTERS:

◆ Try to keep your hips stationary. Imagine that your body is segmented and the parts can move separately.

◆ Reach your arms out as far as you can and as close to shoulder height as you can, but don't obsess about your "form."

◆ Use the knee-bend to exaggerate the stretch along your rib cage and hip.

ARM AND TORSO LENGTHENING

I especially love this exercise because its gestures are flowing, feminine, and free. One of my students told me it brought out the little girl in her since it reminded her of her childhood ballet class. Give yourself permission to engage your whole body and spirit as you perform Arm and Torso Lengthening. Think of healing, expanding, and breathing deeply into the movements.

You are going to perform two sets of the same arm movements. But your feet are going to change position in the middle of the exercise. Shifting your feet trains your body to locate your center of balance.

WHAT YOU NEED FOR THIS EXERCISE: A supporting chair.

STARTING POSITION 1: Stand with the chair to your left and hold on to it with your left hand. Place your heels together and turn your toes out slightly. (In ballet this is known as "first position.") You may also point your toes forward if that is more comfortable. Your right arm hangs just slightly in front of you.

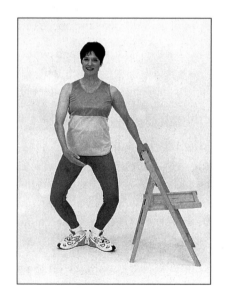

COUNTS: Each set of arm movements takes eight beats.

STEP 1: Slowly bend your knees out to the sides and over your feet. Lift your upper body as you bend your knees, as if your head where attached to a string from the ceiling. This will give you a feeling of stretch through your upper torso. Then, as you begin to straighten them, bring your right arm forward and up in an arc until it's over your head. If your arm can't go this high because you feel pain, that's okay. Bring your arm only as high as is comfortable. Allow your eyes and head to follow your hand while you do the arm movements. This gives the muscles of your neck a stretch as well as your arm and shoulder—and it is a lovely, feminine gesture.

STEP 2: At the top of your arc, turn your wrist so your palm now faces the ceiling—as if you were holding a tray high in the air. Flex your wrist. Feel a stretch from your inner wrist all the way down the inside of your arm to your armpit. (Some women also feel this stretch in their shoulders.)

STEP 3: Next, slowly move your arm straight out and down to the right keeping your hand flexed. Your fingers will trail. Continue circling it all the way back to the starting position. Relax your hand for a moment.

Repeat. Then turn around so you are standing with the chair to your right. Switch arms and do the exercise two times on your left side. When you have finished, turn around and immediately go on to Starting Position 2.

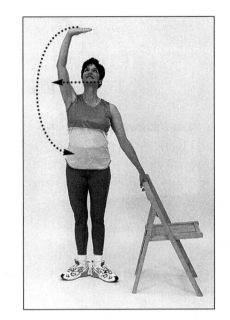

STARTING POSITION 2: Stand with the chair to your left and hold on to it with your left hand. Place your feet hip-width apart. (In ballet this is known as "second position.") Your toes may point forward or slightly outward, whichever stance feels natural. Your weight should be distributed equally between the right and left sides of your body. Imagine you're on a boat in a turbulent ocean and you don't want to get knocked over.

STEP 1: Slowly bend your knees. As you straighten them, repeat the same sequence of arm and head movements as you did in Starting Position 1.

Do two sets of arm movements with your right arm and two with your left arm.

ADVANCED ARM AND TORSO LENGTHENING FOR BOTH ARMS: Once you've advanced to a full range of motion without pain, and you feel confident about your balance, you may choose to work both arms at once. Please realize, however, that it may take several months before you can achieve this goal.

When you have progressed to this level, do three repetitions of your arm movements from Starting Position 1 and three repetitions from Starting Position 2.

POINTERS:

◆ Don't worry if you can't achieve the full arc. You will in time. When you feel pain—as opposed to stretching—stop and pull back a tiny bit. This is your range of motion for now. Work right there.

◆ If you find that doing two repetitions on each side is too difficult, do it once. Please remember, exercise is a lifetime project. You are the one who sets the pace.

◆ If your muscles tire, then stop and rest.

LARGE ARM CIRCLES TO THE FRONT

Even as a five-year survivor, I have learned that my scar tissue gets tighter when I don't do my Large Arm Circles at least three times a week and I lose some of my range of motion. These circles expand the chest wall, strengthen the arm and shoulder muscles, and also improve balance.

COUNTS: Each circle takes eight beats.

STARTING POSITION: Stand with your feet ten to twelve inches apart. Or sit upright in a chair, with your back and neck comfortably straight. Check your posture. Place your right arm straight out in front of you. If you can lift it enough, begin with your arm overhead.

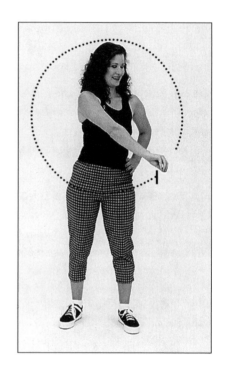

STEP 1: Pretend there's a blackboard in front of you and you're holding a piece of chalk. Slowly draw a large circle going clockwise. Follow your hands with your head. Your goal is to draw as big a circle as possible at your current arm level. Make two. When you're finished, shake out your right arm and relax your muscles.

STEP 2: Switch arms and make two circles on the left, going clockwise. Begin and end with your left arm overhead or directly in front of you. Then shake your left arm out.

STEP 3: Switch arms again, and reverse direction. Your right arm circles counterclockwise twice. Shake it out. Your left arm circles counterclockwise twice. Shake it out.

POINTERS:

◆ Make sure your chest is facing directly forward during the whole exercise.

◆ Don't be discouraged if you can't do a complete circle right away. You are as flexible as you can be today; the more you practice the more flexible you'll become. A seventy-three-year-old survivor in my class could only make small ovals at first. Still, she persisted and in a couple of months could draw the full circle.

LARGE ARM CIRCLES TO THE SIDE

Large Arm Circles to the Side are a continuation of the previous exercise.

STARTING POSITION: Your imaginary chalkboard is now on your right side. Keep your chest facing directly frontward. Lift your right arm in front of you, or take it straight up overhead. The human anatomy doesn't actually allow the arm to move straight back, so your new circles will be drawn a short distance away from the body.

COUNTS: Each circle takes eight beats.

STEP 1: Circle your right arm up and back as far as you can. Slowly continue moving it down, then forward, and back up. Make two circles. Shake out your right arm.

STEP 2: Switch arms. Make two circles with your left arm moving backward. Shake out your left arm.

STEP 3: Then reverse direction. Make two forward circles with your right arm. Shake it out. Switch to the left arm and make two forward circles. Shake out your left arm.

You are now sufficiently stretched and ready to perform one of the exercise programs targeted to a specific issue in Part Two, "Adjusting to the Needs of Your New Body," the Ultimate Movements in Part Three, or a sports warm-up from Part Four. Good luck and have fun!

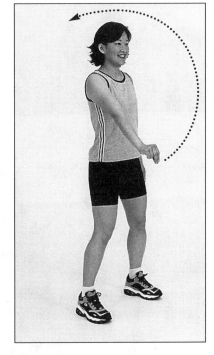

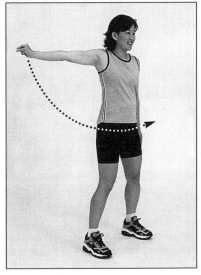

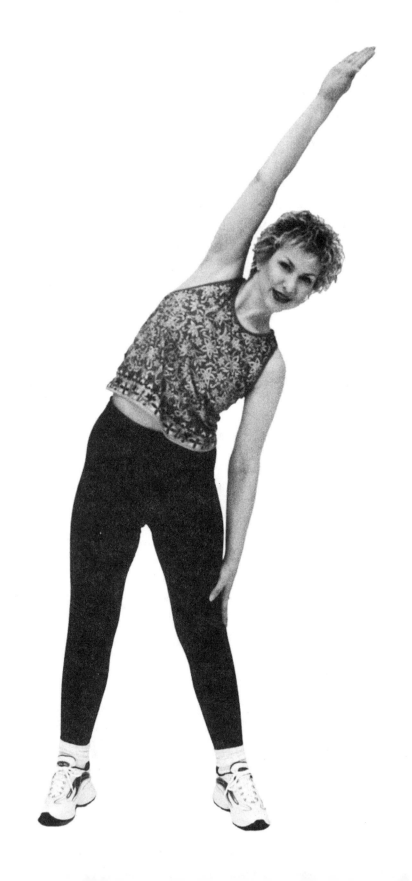

PART TWO

Adjusting to the Needs
of
Your New Body

As a breast cancer survivor, your body has changed. You have undergone surgery and possibly radiation therapy, chemotherapy, or both. As a result, you have some different needs than you once did. While it is true that everyone responds in her own way to treatment and has an individual pattern of recovery, there are also certain issues that many of us face both in the short term and in the long term. Our physical challenges can include pain, fatigue, loss of range of motion, and difficulty balancing, among others. Our emotional challenges can include such things as recovering a sense of femininity and libido or coping with anger, depression, and mood swings. No matter what the issue is, exercise can be an effective way of handling it.

The exercise programs in Part Two, "Adjusting to the Needs of Your New Body," are targeted to the kinds of challenges you may face during and after your surgery and other treatments. I have arranged them in the sequence in which they generally come up. They cover:

◆ Restoring Flexibility
◆ Moving Through Pain
◆ Combating Fatigue
◆ Emotional Recovery
◆ Living with Lymphedema
◆ Developing Balance
◆ Menopause
◆ Exploring Your Femininity
◆ After Reconstruction

Since you know better than anyone how your body feels at any given moment, you are the best judge of which program you need to follow. It is, however, unlikely that you are going to need to work on all of these programs. When deciding which to do, I recommend that you read the section in the introduction of each chapter labeled "Specifics for Survivors" and consider the guidelines and precautions it mentions.

Every chapter in Part Two contains a program of exercises targeting your upper and lower body, followed by a dance routine and healing visualization. The exception is "Emotional Recovery," which includes two meditations instead of a healing visualization. Feel free to exchange and play around with the different visualizations and meditations. They are designed to be interchangeable. You should always precede these workouts by doing the Basic Warm-up. I encourage you to perform the program of your choice at least three times a week.

Your primary goal right now should be to restore your complete range of motion and become pain-free. Afterward, you can work on the routines that address your other areas of concern, such as lymphedema, balance, or menopause. When these needs have been resolved, you will be ready to move on to Part Three, "The Ultimate Movements." This is a maintenance routine you can do for the rest of your life. In the meantime, your secondary goal should be to keep moving and get stronger. You may also find that you enjoy the Part Two targeted programs so much that you'll want to return to them occasionally in order to add variety to your workout schedule.

RESTORING FLEXIBILITY

"I had no mobility before Focus on Healing. It had been six years and my
shoulder was frozen. The arm on the side where my surgery was done
simply did not lift as high as it used to. Movement was not only limited, it
also hurt. After doing these exercises, I have full range of motion, no
frozen shoulder, and no more pain."

—*Denise, forty-eight*

The most common problem faced by women who have had breast cancer surgery is the loss of flexibility. This is true no matter what kind of surgery you have undergone. Flexibility depends on the elasticity of the muscles and scar tissue in your chest and arm. Scar tissue tightens and pulls in as it develops, limiting your range of motion. In addition, radiation therapy is known to shrink and toughen skin and underlying tissue. It is extremely important to stretch regularly to soften your scar tissue, and to prevent your muscles from contracting severely. This should be a lifelong practice.

When your range of motion decreases, you may find yourself unable to do the everyday actions that you normally would not think twice about. It can interfere with something as simple as getting dressed and tying your shoes. The longer you remain immobile after surgery the more the lack of flexibility can become a problem. So it is critical to begin stretching as soon as possible after surgery and your drain is removed—even within a matter of days—and often while you are still feeling pain and fatigue.

At fifty-six, Mary was a one-year survivor of breast cancer when I met her. Her hospital had advertised the Focus on Healing program in its newsletter and she phoned me with some questions. She told me she'd had difficulty with her range of motion ever since the surgery, but at the time her main concern had been to get through all her treatments and survive. She was a retired real estate agent, lived with her husband, saw her grandkids on the weekends, and did some light gardening. She had thought that her stiffness was an inevitable sign of aging and that she'd just have to take some painkillers and cope. Recently, however, she'd been focusing more closely on what was going wrong with her arm and realized it was getting worse.

It had never crossed Mary's mind that her condition could be a result of her surgery. She thought she was supposed to be healed. She had been resting her arm thinking her pain and stiffness were symptoms of something else, such as bursitis. In fact, even as we spoke, she reiterated her confidence that it wasn't from the surgery. But she wondered if my program could help her anyway. I told her, "You can't lose anything by coming in and trying the program and seeing how it feels."

After our conversation, Mary came to my class once a week and also did the exercises on her own at home three to four times a week. Once she saw that there was something she could do to correct her physical problem, she became very determined to improve her situation. Her success was not only due to the program itself but to her determination and willingness to do the program often at home, constantly keeping at it. To me, this was a sign of her incredible courageousness.

The worst-case scenario in terms of decreased flexibility is an extreme condition known as frozen shoulder. This is the name for a collection of multiple underlying conditions that lead to a common outcome—a painful rotator cuff with limited motion. Your arm literally becomes locked into the wrong position. Too many women don't understand that frozen shoulder can occur as a complication of surgery and radiation even years later. Since moving the shoulder causes pain, survivors start to believe that not moving their arm and shoulder is the right thing to do. But it's not. The longer you don't use your arm after surgery the worse your frozen shoulder can get.

One of the best means anyone has yet found to restore flexibility is through gentle stretching. Stretching through your complete range of motion can actually help break up scar tissue, which then is reabsorbed into the body. It is never too late to regain your flexibility.

FLEXIBILITY SPECIFICS FOR SURVIVORS You should practice the "Restoring Flexibility" routine until you have regained your complete range of motion, which is defined as the ability to reach your arm straight overhead and bring it back until it's slightly behind your ear. Once you have achieved this goal, you are ready to move on to the other routines in Part Two that address significant issues of concern, such as balance, or continue further on to the Ultimate Movements in Part Three.

Three of the exercises in this routine incorporate the use of an elastic exercise band without handles. *Caution:* Never wrap the ends of the band around your hands; this can cut off your circulation and trigger lymphedema, a persistent swelling.

Please remember to do your stretches gently. Imagine that your muscles and scar tissue are like rubber bands. If you quickly pull a rubber band to the end of its resistance, it is going to snap back. But if you take it and pull it gently and slowly, you are going to get more distance out of it and more elasticity. That elasticity is healthy flexibility. So relax and breathe deeply as you gently coax your muscles into the stretch.

THE RESTORING FLEXIBILITY ROUTINE

- The Basic Warm-up (p. 15–23)
- Mountain High Stretch
- Wall Push-ups
- The Crawl
- The Backstroke
- The Breaststroke
- Arm Rotations
- Single-Arm Reach
- Climbing the Ladder
- Close-the-Door Lunges
- Circle the Moon
- Yawn Stretch
- Bicep Curl
- Shoulder Blade Contraction
- Dance Routine
- Healing Visualization

MOUNTAIN HIGH STRETCH

Begin here, after doing the Basic Warm-up. This stretch gently elongates your scar tissue and helps prevent frozen shoulder. If you cannot bring your arms overhead yet, bring them as high as you can in front of your body.

STARTING POSITION: Stand with your feet hip-width apart, your arms hanging by your sides.

STEP 1: Bring both arms forward and up, until they are overhead. Hook your fingers together and turn the palms of your hands up to the ceiling. Pull your shoulders up toward your ears. Inhale as you stretch up.

STEP 2: Keeping your fingers interlaced, press your shoulders down hard. Exhale. Repeat steps 1 and 2 four times.

STEP 3: Next, still keeping your fingers interlaced, tilt your body to the right. Hold and breathe deeply.

STEP 4: Come upright again and tilt to the left. Hold and breathe deeply.

STEP 5: Come upright again and unhook your fingers. With your wrists flexed, slowly lower your arms out to the sides and return them to the starting position.

Do two complete sets.

POINTER:

◆ Keep your elbows as straight as possible when your fingers are interlocked.

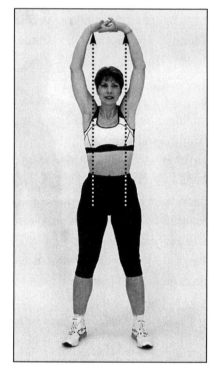

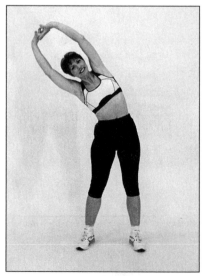

WALL PUSH-UPS

Wall Push-ups are an easy way to open up your chest, build arm strength, and increase your range of motion. You may either do them in the corner of a room, which is optimum, or facing a flat wall.

STARTING POSITION: Stand two feet away from the wall with your legs hip-width apart. Place your arms at chest height on the wall and your hands about a foot apart. If this is an uncomfortable distance, move closer. For a greater chest stretch, move your hands farther apart. Turn your fingers slightly toward each other. If this position hurts your wrists, find a compensating position that suits your special needs. Turn your hands as upright as necessary to eliminate any wrist discomfort.

COUNTS: Every Wall Push-up takes four counts.

STEP 1: On a slow count of two, bend your arms and lean into the wall, bringing your face about four inches away from it. Be careful not to sway your back or cave in. Your body should be as straight as a wooden board.

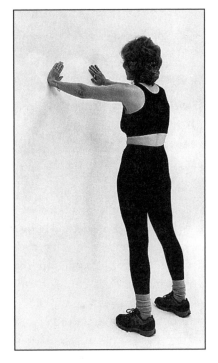

STEP 2: Push back on another count of two to return to the starting position.

Begin with two push-ups. Then gradually increase the number you're doing from two to twelve over the course of a month or two. Whenever you feel strong enough to do more repetitions, add two push-ups. You should stay at the same level for at least three more workouts before adding on again.

POINTERS:

◆ Stop if you feel pain in your arms. You can relieve some of the strain on your arms by lifting your elbows and turning your fingertips to face each other.

◆ Concentrate on tightening your buttocks.

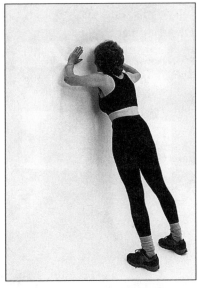

THE CRAWL

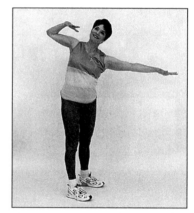

The Crawl helps to stretch out the muscles and scar tissue along your sides. It also improves your shoulder rotation and loosens your neck. The best things about "swimming" on dry land are that it won't mess up your makeup and no hairdryer is needed!

STARTING POSITION: Stand with your feet hip-width apart. Your arms should be straight out in front of your body at shoulder height—or as high as you can lift them.

COUNTS: Every arm circle takes eight counts.

STEP 1: To do the Crawl, your arms must cycle independently. Lower your right arm down to your side, then bend your right elbow, and bring the arm up to shoulder height. From shoulder height, continue the movement by extending the arm straight up in the air.

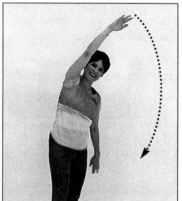

STEP 2: At the same time, bring your left arm down to your side, then bend the left elbow and bring your left arm up to shoulder height. As the left arm is rising, circle the right arm forward and down to the starting position. As the left arm continues straight up into the air, lower your right arm to your side.

Circle both arms four times. Turn your head to the right as your right hand reaches your shoulder and then turn it to the left as your left hand reaches your shoulder. Your movements should be continuous and flowing. It doesn't matter whether you do this perfectly. The idea is to get your arms working one after the other and find a steady rhythm.

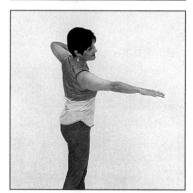

POINTER:
◆ Imagine the resistance of the water.

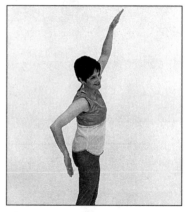

THE BACKSTROKE

To achieve full range of motion you must stretch the muscles of your back as well as your chest. The Backstroke is graceful and gets your blood circulating. One major benefit you'll soon enjoy is being able to reach behind you to grab your seat belt. As you do this exercise, lift your arms only as high as you are able right now. In time you will improve.

STARTING POSITION: Stand with your feet hip-width apart. Place your arms straight in front of your body at shoulder height.

COUNTS: Each arm circle takes four counts.

STEP 1: Keeping your right arm as straight as possible, circle it back and down, and then return it to the starting position.

STEP 2: As your right arm is on its way down, begin making a similar backward circle with your left arm. The two arms will be rotating one after the other like a windmill.

Make four circles with each arm.

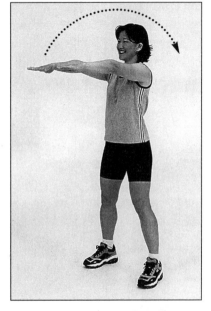

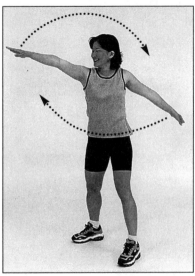

THE BREASTSTROKE

The Breaststroke opens and stretches your entire chest area. Everyday living can be vastly improved by restoring your range of motion out to the sides and backward. These movements were a great confidence booster for me during my recovery. At first I could only reach part of the way back, but then, over several months, I regained a full range of movement.

STARTING POSITION: Stand with your feet hip-width apart and your knees slightly bent. Bring your hands together in front of your chest at shoulder height and let your elbows come up and out to the side. Your palms are facing front. Lean forward a tiny bit and look straight ahead.

COUNTS: Each Breaststroke takes four beats. Every arm movement is one count.

STEP 1: Push your palms forward, keeping them at shoulder height.

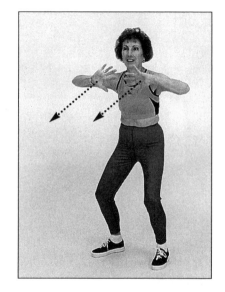

STEP 2: When your arms are fully extended in front of you, circle them out to your sides and simultaneously straighten your legs.

STEP 3: Keeping your legs straight, drop your arms to your sides. Then bend your knees and return to the starting position.
 Repeat four times.

POINTERS:

◆ Be sure to spread your arms wide to the side to feel the expanse of the stretch across your chest.

◆ This is a great exercise for breathing. Inhale as you move your arms forward and exhale as you return to the starting position.

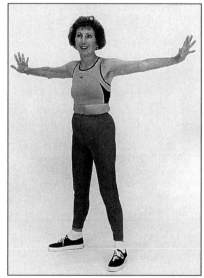

ARM ROTATIONS

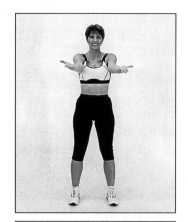

*"I am thrilled with my increase in range of motion.
I can reach higher and have more strength."*
—BEV, SIXTY-THREE

This exercise rotates your armpits and shoulders to help prevent and get rid of frozen shoulder.

STARTING POSITION: Stand with your feet hip-width apart. Your arms are extended out in front of you at chest height, palms facing the ceiling. Your elbows remain straight throughout this program.

COUNTS: Every movement takes two counts.

STEP 1: Turn your palms inward to face each other.

STEP 2: Then turn them downward.

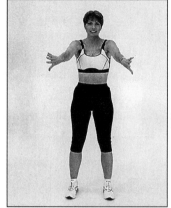

STEP 3: Turn them outward so that the backs of your hands face each other.

STEP 4: Then turn them downward again.

STEP 5: Turn them inward.

STEP 6: Then turn them upward again to the starting position.
Repeat four times.

STEP 7: Next, move your arms out to the sides at shoulder height with your palms still facing the ceiling.

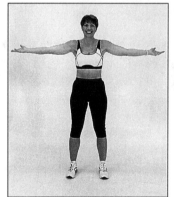

STEP 8: Turn them forward.

STEP 9: Then turn them downward.

STEP 10: Turn them backward.

STEP 11: Then turn them up, allowing your shoulder to roll forward.

STEP 12: Reverse direction and turn them backward again.

STEP 13: Turn them downward.

STEP 14: Turn them frontward.

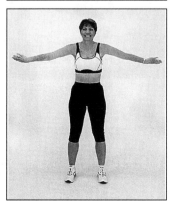

STEP 15: Then turn them upward again.
Repeat four times.

SINGLE-ARM REACH

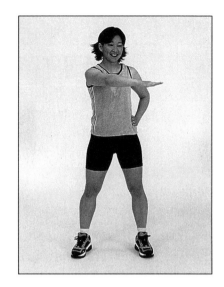

You will feel this stretch across the top of your back, below your shoulder blades, and across your rib cage. It has a similar feeling to a dog pulling eagerly on the end of a leash. The resistance you provide is what makes the stretch happen.

STARTING POSITION: Stand with your feet hip-width apart. Your left hand is on your hip.

STEP 1: Raise your right arm to shoulder height. Then move it to the left across your chest. Keep your right arm straight. Reach your right arm farther to the left as though someone were pulling your arm and saying "Come with me!" Resist with your right shoulder, as though you were responding "No, I don't want to go!" and pulling back. Then release the tension.

Do four stretches with your right arm.

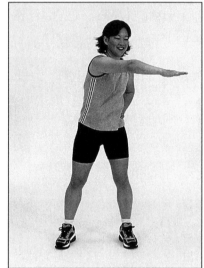

STEP 2: Reverse your arms. Repeat the stretch four times with your left arm.

POINTERS:

◆ Keep your arms straight.

◆ Keep your hips facing front.

CLIMBING THE LADDER

"By climbing the ladder, I can reach higher and have much more strength. And it's fun."
—AMELIA, THIRTY-NINE

You may already be familiar with this exercise, as most survivors are given some variation of it when they are discharged from the hospital. A pumping action has been added in this version to increase your circulation.

STARTING POSITION: Stand with your feet hip-width apart. Make loose fists with your hands and place them at your waist.

COUNTS: Every movement takes two counts.

STEP 1: First, reach your right arm forward at waist height. Open your hand, bring your right shoulder forward, and bend your right knee, shifting your weight to your right leg.

STEP 2: Now reach your left arm forward at waist height, bend your left knee, bring your left shoulder forward, and open your left hand. Your weight shifts to your left leg. At the same time, straighten your right knee and pull your right hand back in to your waist, making a fist again.

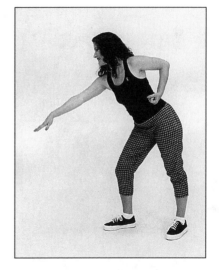

STEP 3: Reverse the arms, shoulders, and legs again—reaching your right hand forward to *shoulder height*, with your left hand coming back to your waist, where you make a fist.

STEP 4: Reverse the movements again. Reach your left arm out to *shoulder height* and pull your right hand back to your waist and make a fist.

STEP 5: Reverse the movements again. This time, though, reach your right arm forward to *face height*. Pull your left hand back to your waist.

STEP 6: Then do the reverse with your left arm to *face height* and your right arm coming into your waist.

STEP 7: For the next four beats, alternate reaching *above your head* first with the right arm and then with the left arm, bending the same knee as the arm that is reaching upward. Continue

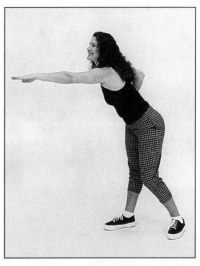

opening your hand as your arm reaches full extension and closing your hand as it comes down to your waist.

STEP 8: Now repeat the same actions you made going up, this time moving downward. First reach your hands to *face height*, then reach them to *shoulder height*, and finally to *waist height*.

Complete two whole series.

POINTERS:

◆ This series of movements must be performed slowly to protect you from injury.

◆ Imagine that you are squeezing two rubber balls as you open and close your fists.

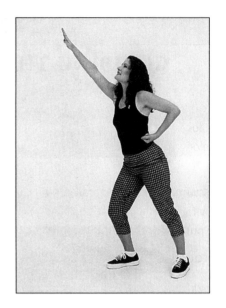

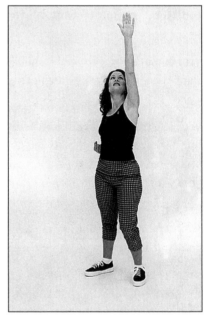

CLOSE-THE-DOOR LUNGES

Close-the-Door Lunges stretch the scar tissue and tendons along your arm from your wrist to your armpit. Your legs can also get a good workout.

STARTING POSITION: Stand with your feet together. Make a fist with your right hand and bend your arm so that your fist is by your shoulder, as if you're going to box with someone.

COUNTS: Every lunge takes four counts.

STEP 1: Keeping your left leg stationary, lunge your right leg forward about three feet, bending your right knee. As you lunge, your right arm shoots forward and your right hand opens to a flexed position, as if you're slamming a door shut.

STEP 2: Then push off your right heel and bring your leg back to the starting position. At the same time, retract your arm and clench your hand into a fist again.

Do four lunges on the right.

Switch arms and repeat the same series four times on the left.

POINTERS:

◆ Imagine that the door you are slamming is moving farther away from you so that each time your arm goes out farther. This increases the stretch across your upper shoulders and back.

◆ Flex the wrist of your extended arm as much as possible in the lunge position.

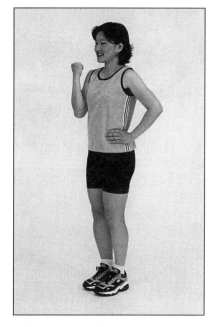

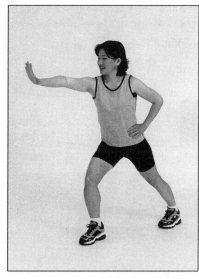

CIRCLE THE MOON

Circle the Moon works your full range of motion. Make as large a circle as you can, even if it's only a small oval—increase the size of your circle when you are able. Allow yourself to experience how graceful the movement can be.

STARTING POSITION: Stand with your feet hip-width apart, and your arms hanging by your sides.

COUNTS: Every circle takes eight counts.

STEP 1: Both arms move together. Imagine that you're holding a small beach ball between your hands. Circle them to the right, then up overhead, and then down on the left. Repeat.
  Then circle your arms twice in the opposite direction.

POINTER:
◆ Move very slowly.

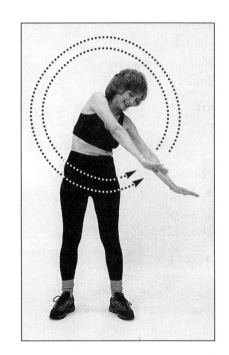

YAWN STRETCH

The next three exercises use an elastic exercise band without handles to strengthen and tone your muscles. The Yawn Stretch works your back, shoulder area, and upper arms. When I do this movement first thing in the morning, I find that I don't feel as stiff and sore during the day.

WHAT YOU NEED FOR THIS EXERCISE: An elastic exercise band without handles; a chair is optional.

STARTING POSITION: Sit or stand with your feet hip-width apart. Extend your arms over your head and hold your elastic band in an overhanded grip. Your hands are spread about a foot and a half apart. Keep your elbows straight. If you cannot lift your arms overhead yet, raise them as high as possible and do the stretch at this height.

COUNTS: Four counts to open and four counts to close.

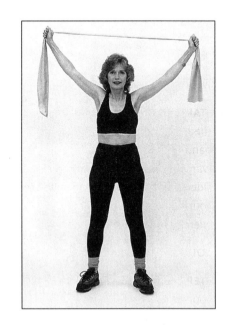

STEP 1: Spread your arms open and back as far as you can, as if you are having a huge yawn. Keep your arms straight and bring your hands as close to shoulder level as possible. Inhale deeply. The band should run behind your head, if possible.

STEP 2: Then bring your hands back up to the starting position. Exhale.

Do four Yawn Stretches.

POINTERS:

◆ Watch out for your hair. When it gets caught in the band it can be a nightmare to untangle. The best thing is to tie your hair back in a ponytail.

◆ Move slowly!

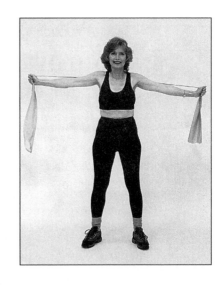

FLEXIBILITY 12

BICEP CURL

Bicep Curls work your chest and the upper and lower parts of your arms. You should notice your strength returning and your body being energized after doing these for only a few weeks.

WHAT YOU NEED FOR THIS EXERCISE: An elastic exercise band.

STARTING POSITION: Step on one end of your band, either with the heel or the ball of your right foot. Hold the other end of the band in your right hand. The palm of your hand is turned forward, and the end of your band dangles from the little finger side of your fist. Lock your right arm tight against the side of your body. Your wrist should be straight, not flexed during this exercise and you should stand tall.

COUNTS: Four counts to curl and four counts to release.

STEP 1: Bend your right elbow and slowly bring your hand up to your shoulder. Return slowly to the starting position. Repeat four times.

STEP 2: Switch the elastic band to your left hand and foot. When you are ready, repeat the Bicep Curl four times with your left arm.

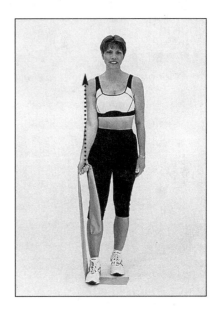

POINTER:

◆ I find that I have more balance and strength when I put the foot on my working side a little bit behind the other. But this is a matter of preference. You should take the stance that is most comfortable for you.

SHOULDER BLADE CONTRACTION

The outward and inward movements of the Shoulder Blade Contraction are equally important as you are using two different sets of muscles to perform each. As you master this exercise you will regain a sense of control.

WHAT YOU NEED FOR THIS EXERCISE: An elastic exercise band; a chair is optional.

STARTING POSITION: Stand or sit with your feet hip-width apart. Check your posture. Hold the band in a loose overhanded grip near your chest. Palms should face down, and wrist should be straight, not flexed. Your hands are about a foot and a half apart. Your elbows are lifted to shoulder height.

COUNTS: Four counts to extend and four counts to return.

STEP 1: Straighten your arms slowly out to the sides. Feel your shoulder blades pull together and your chest expand forward.

STEP 2: Then slowly bend your elbows and return your hands to the starting position.
    Repeat four times.

POINTER:
◆ Don't arch your back.

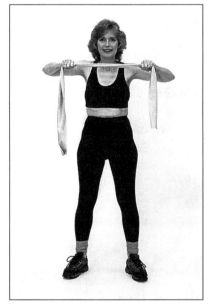

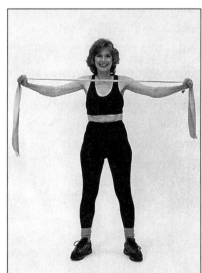

DANCE ROUTINE

"As the music swells to a crescendo, my pain symptoms disappear. I shimmy and kick through the entire song and it feels so good. I find I have a greater range of motion—without the pain."
—SIMONE, FIFTY-SEVEN

Now it's time to have fun and move freely. You are thoroughly warmed up from the previous exercises and your joints are lubricated and flexible. The pleasure of dancing can help you go beyond your physical and emotional limitations.

MUSICAL SUGGESTION: Ricky Martin, "She Bangs."

STARTING POSITION: Stand with your feet together; your arms hanging by your sides.

STEP-DRAG: Step out to the side with your right foot and bring your right arm overhead. At the same time, extend your left arm to the side. Then drag your left foot slowly toward the right foot, while lowering your arms. Rest lightly on the ball of your left foot.

Then step out to the side with your left foot, and bring your left arm overhead. At the same time, extend your right arm to the side. Drag the right foot slowly toward the left foot, while lowering your arms. Rest lightly on the ball of your right foot.

Repeat the series. Then go on to Step-Touches.

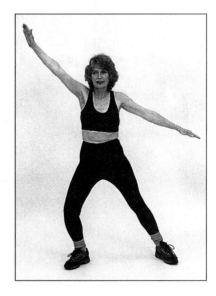

STEP-TOUCH: Step to the right, swinging your arms up and to the right. Then touch your left foot to the side and clap your hands at the same time. Step to the left, swinging your arms up and to the left. Touch your right foot to the side and clap your hands at the same time.

Do eight sets.

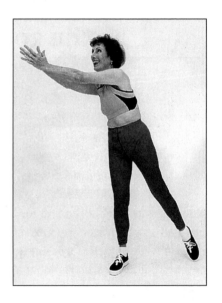

THE SHOWGIRL STRUT: Step to the right, swinging your arms from left to right overhead like a Las Vegas showgirl with attitude. Then touch your left foot to the side. Step to the left, swinging your arms overhead from right to left. Then touch your right foot to the side.

Do eight sets.

Then come to a stationary position in preparation for Arm Flops. Stand with your feet hip-width apart and your arms down at your sides

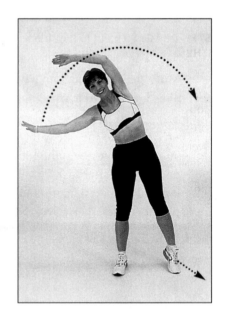

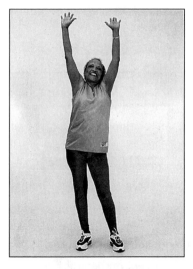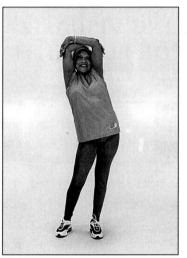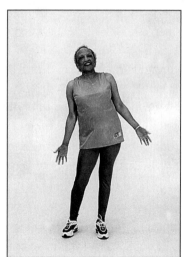

ARM FLOPS: Reach your arms up, and then flop them down behind your head. Reach them up again, and flop them down to your sides. Swing your hips from right to left while doing your arm movements.

Do four times, and then move on to the Hawaiian Hula.

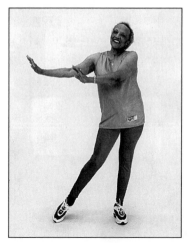

THE HAWAIIAN HULA: Step out to the right with your right foot, and then bring your left foot to join it, letting your hips sway in an exaggerated motion. Step to the right again, and touch the ball of your left foot next to it. As you take your steps, brush the air to the right with the backs of your hands as if they were flowing through water.

Now travel left, stepping out to the left and bringing your right foot to join it with the same hand gesture.

Repeat the series.

Do the whole routine from beginning to end as many times as possible until the song ends. Then walk slowly around the room for one minute, or walk in place, to lower your heart rate. Breathe deeply in and out to feed your body with oxygen and take a drink of water.

Now spend a few quiet minutes doing the Healing Visualization that follows.

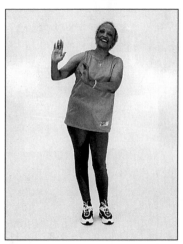

HEALING VISUALIZATION
FOR FLEXIBILITY

Sit down in a chair in a comfortable position and close your eyes. Slowly tune in to your body. Are your feet, ankles, and legs relaxed? How about your hands, wrists, and arms? Do you feel any tightness in your upper body? How about your face? Allow your jaw and the muscles in your back, shoulders, and neck to release. Sometimes becoming aware of tension is all it takes to relax. Be with yourself in this moment. Accept yourself as you are—just for now.

Take long, deep breaths in through your nose and out through your mouth. Visualize a warm golden light enveloping your body like a nurturing embrace. Every breath makes it grow stronger and more tangible.

Imagine that it is a lovely spring day. You are outside running barefoot through a vast field or some other favorite place in nature. You can smell the moist earth and greenness of the new plants. You can feel the grass between your toes. There is nothing holding you back from skipping, climbing a tree, or doing a cartwheel. In this special place you have absolutely no limitations.

Say three times, "I accept my body as it is today and feel it growing freer and more expansive."

When you are done playing and feel ready, open your eyes and come back.

MOVING THROUGH PAIN

"Dealing with the loss of my breasts and treatment two years ago was very difficult, and then I also found myself losing the use of my arms and range of motion. Simple tasks were becoming very painful and almost impossible to accomplish. No one in the medical field had any answers for me and I felt that my quality of life, as I knew it, was over. After doing the Focus on Healing exercises I slowly began to improve, until now I have full range of motion and no more pain."

—*Pat, fifty-six*

*P*ain is perhaps the most significant quality of life issue that a breast cancer survivor must face. It can interfere with your ability to perform ordinary tasks like fastening a seat belt, brushing your teeth, reaching into a high cabinet, and hugging your children. It can distract you while you are working and prevent you from getting a good night's sleep. For so many reasons, it is both physically and emotionally draining. The good news is that exercise truly helps survivors manage and alleviate all kinds of pain.

Linda, fifty-one, is a two-year survivor who had a bilateral mastectomy. Before doing Focus on Healing, her shoulders and neck constantly ached. Every night she had to take a large dose of ibuprofen before bed. Her doctor believed she had tendonitis because her chest was fully healed. Even though Linda was initially skeptical, the very first time she did this exercise program she was able to stop taking medication. She then became a regular participant and moved on to address other issues that were troubling her, such as her balance.

Debbie, thirty-five, is a stay-at-home mom who home schools her three young children and volunteers for an animal rights organization. She regularly does Focus on Healing to control her chronic pain. Four months after completing radiation, intense pain pulsed from her shoulder down her right side and arm. Her doctor wisely identified the source of the problem as the scar tissue from her surgery and radiation, and gave her a flyer for a class on this program. Now Debbie is pain-free most of the time and understands that stretching is what eases her discomfort. The exercises she learned enable her to maintain an active lifestyle and honor the commitments she has made to her family and community.

Breast cancer survivors feel pain for many different reasons. Painful sensations may be located in your shoulder, neck, chest, upper or lower back, arm, or along your side anywhere from the underarm to the hip. Postsurgical pain is typically sharp at first and then fades to tenderness. Years later, pain may be connected to other physical issues like frozen shoulder, arthritis, or bursitis. Sometimes pain is dull. It can come from overdoing an activity such as riding a bike or gardening, or even from sleeping in an odd position. Oftentimes the source is tough scar tissue or muscles fibers that were shortened by radiation and surgery. No matter what the cause, pain is not a punishment, although it may occasionally feel like one. Rather, it is a message your body is sending that something needs your attention.

PAIN SPECIFICS FOR SURVIVORS Before you address any other issue you may be facing, I strongly suggest that you practice the exercise routine in this chapter and get a handle on your pain. The one exception is when lymphedema is the source of your discomfort. In that case, first turn to "Living with Lymphedema" (p. 88) and work on the exercises there. Return to this chapter if you are still experiencing pain after your swelling has been reduced. Once your pain goes away or significantly abates, you are ready to move on to the other chapters in Part Three that address specific topics of concern, such as flexibility, fatigue, and emotional recovery, or shift to the Ultimate Movements in Part Three.

The exercise routine here is designed to help ease the pain you are experiencing by stretching your scar tissue and muscle fibers, building correct body placement, and releasing natural painkillers called endorphins into your bloodstream. While you are doing these movements, I want you to pay close attention to your breath as well as your body. Taking long, deep inhalations as you thoughtfully perform the movements will assist you in moving through your pain.

One of your goals is to extend your capacity to move. Yet only you can determine whether you are pushing yourself too far beyond your current limits. The way to assess this is by noticing and responding to your internal sensations. Here's a rule of thumb I offer in my classes: If your pain increases rather than decreases during the range of any movement, stop and return to the point before the excess pain began. That is exactly where you want to work. It may take a little time for you to feel confident, so until then being cautious is appropriate. I would rather you do what you feel you can safely do and then build on your successes.

If your pain feels too severe to comfortably stand and move, then do this routine in a chair.

Conserve your energy for the arm movements. In any case, you should perform the Basic Warm-up routine very slowly while seated.

THE MOVING THROUGH PAIN ROUTINE
- The Basic Warm-up (pp. 15–23)
- Hanging Spirals
- Big Hug
- Flying Angels
- Olympic Weight Lifting
- Leg Lifts
- Calf and Leg Builder
- Leg Pendulums
- Dance Routine
- Healing Visualization

HANGING SPIRALS

Begin here, after doing the Basic Warm-up. The purpose of this seated exercise is to increase the circulation in your arm, arm sockets, and shoulders.

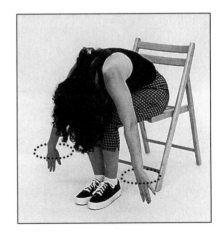

WHAT YOU NEED FOR THIS EXERCISE: A chair.

STARTING POSITION: Sit all the way back in your chair with your knees close together and your feet flat on the floor.

STEP 1: Roll your upper body slowly forward, until your head and arms are dangling toward your feet, as though you were trying to recover from a faint. First, bend your head forward until your chin touches your chest. Then let your shoulders cave in. Then the rest of the spine starts rounding down, one vertebra at a time. Hold at the bottom, bending forward at the hips and leaning your chest against your thighs. Your arms and head are dangling forward.

STEP 2: Now make small circles above the floor with both your hands, four times in one direction and then four times in the opposite direction. Repeat.

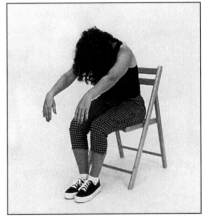

STEP 3: Slowly roll up through your spine. As you come up, bring your arms up in front of your body and then overhead.

STEP 4: Flex your wrists so that your palms are facing the ceiling and your fingertips are pointing inward. Keeping your wrists flexed, slowly lower your arms out to the sides and then down. Relax.

POINTERS:

◆ You may feel fluid rushing into your hands. This is normal.

◆ If either arm feels heavy or tired or in unavoidable pain, stop.

◆ If you have any difficulty rolling up, feel free to put your hands on your thighs and give yourself a little leverage.

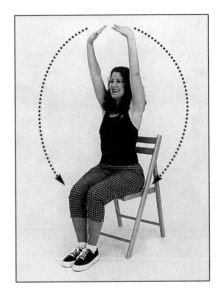

BIG HUG

When we are in pain there is a natural tendency to tighten our muscles to combat it, and then the pain gets worse. Oddly enough, tightening a tense muscle even more deeply and then purposefully relaxing it enables the muscle to release more fully.

WHAT YOU NEED FOR THIS EXERCISE: A chair is optional.

STARTING POSITION: Stand or take a seat, and extend your arms out to your sides at shoulder height.

STEP 1: Wrap your arms around yourself in a Big Hug with your right arm on top.

STEP 2: Extend your arms to the sides again. Then hug yourself with your left arm on top.

Now it is time to get up and move the rest of your body. Walk slowly around the room for a minute, gently swinging your arms from right to left around your body. As you do, make the sound *Aaaahhhh* or let out a long sigh to release your pent-up energy. Then move on to the rest of the exercises.

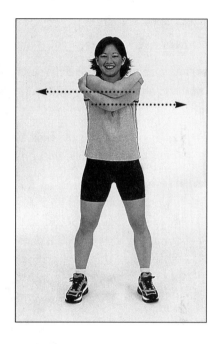

FLYING ANGELS

Did you ever make snow angels when you were a kid? Flying Angels use the same motion, except that you're standing up. It is an excellent and gentle way to stretch out tough scar tissue and release painful shoulders.

STARTING POSITION: Stand with your feet hip-width apart, your arms hanging by your sides, palms flexed.

COUNTS: Every movement takes four counts.

STEP 1: Keeping your palms flexed, lift your arms to the sides and overhead until they are beside your ears. Inhale as you raise your arms.

STEP 2: Then lower your arms. Exhale.
Repeat. As you are able, work up to four Flying Angels.

POINTER:

◆ Only bring your arms high enough to feel a gentle stretch. If that means shoulder height, so be it. Honor the needs of your body as it is today, not as it once was or as you want it to be in the future.

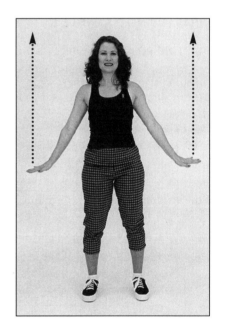

OLYMPIC WEIGHT LIFTING

Don't you just love the Olympics—strong men and women straining under impossibly huge burdens of weights? In this version you create your own "weight" through the amount of resistance you imagine. It can be as hard or as easy as you make it. Not only will your upper body and arms get stronger, you'll also enjoy a terrific stretch along your rib cage, arms, and shoulder.

WHAT YOU NEED FOR THIS EXERCISE: A towel.

STARTING POSITION: Stand with your feet hip-width apart. Hold one end of your towel in each hand with an overhanded grip, and bend your elbows to bring your hands to shoulder height. The towel should be taut.

COUNTS: Every lift takes eight counts. Every side bend takes four.

STEP 1: Take a deep breath in, then push your arms slowly up to the ceiling, creating a resistance in your muscles as if your towel weighs twenty pounds. Exhale on the movement.

STEP 2: Now bring your arms slowly back to the starting position as you inhale, feeling that same resistance.

STEP 3: Do three lifts. On the last lift keep your arms above your head.

STEP 4: Now bend to the right and inhale, keeping the towel taut between your hands. Return to center, exhaling.

STEP 5: Then bend to the left and inhale. Return to the center, exhaling. Bring your arms down to the starting position, and drop the towel.

You may repeat the series when you feel able.

POINTERS:

◆ Hold your stomach in. Don't arch your back.

◆ Only lift as far as you are comfortable.

◆ Keep your head level.

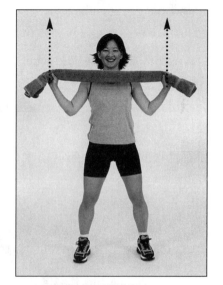

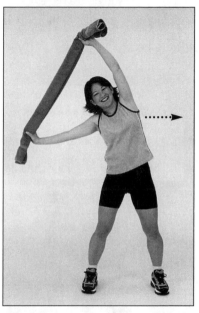

LEG LIFTS

As your center of gravity, the lower body is the foundation of your balance and posture. Therefore you want it to be strong and toned. The next three exercises are done using a supporting chair, and they target your legs, buttocks, and hips.

WHAT YOU NEED FOR THIS EXERCISE: A supporting chair.

STARTING POSITION: Place the chair on your left side and hold on to it with your left hand.

COUNTS: Every movement takes two counts.

STEP 1: Lift your right leg out in front of you about six inches off the floor. Hold for four counts. Lower.

STEP 2: Then lift your right leg out to the side. Hold for four counts. Lower.

STEP 3: Lift your right leg to the back. Hold for four counts. Lower.

STEP 4: Lift your right leg out to the side again. Hold for four counts. Lower.

STEP 5: Now place the chair to your right. Repeat the series with your left leg.

Each time you hold a Leg Lift, see if you can let go of the chair for a moment and maintain your balance without support.

POINTERS:

◆ Lift your legs no higher than six inches off the floor.

◆ Your standing leg should be held straight unless you're having pain in the knee, in which case you may bend it slightly.

◆ Tuck your buttocks and lower abdomen slightly forward.

◆ Remember to press your shoulders down.

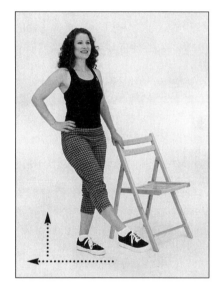

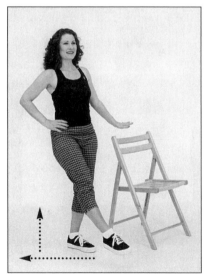

CALF AND LEG BUILDER

What would you be without strong, beautiful legs? How would you stand up or move around? This exercise helps to strengthen your legs so you can center yourself, which in turn will help to relieve neck and shoulder pain.

WHAT YOU NEED FOR THIS EXERCISE: A supporting chair.

STARTING POSITION: Place the chair in front of you and hold on to it with both hands. Stand at arm's length from the chair with your feet together.

COUNTS: Every movement takes one count.

STEP 1: Rise up onto your toes. Come back down. Do eight times.

POINTERS:

◆ Pull in your stomach and tuck your hips slightly forward.

◆ Remember to press your shoulders down.

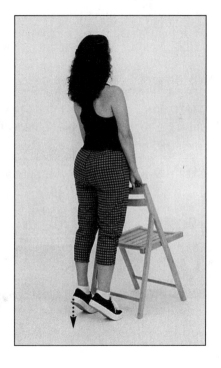

LEG PENDULUMS

All parts of your body are interconnected. Improving your balance and posture with Leg Pendulums can release some of the pain in your back and neck. When I do these movements I experience a sense of flowing and wholeness.

WHAT YOU NEED FOR THIS EXERCISE: A supporting chair.

STARTING POSITION: Place the chair to your left and hold on to it with your left hand. Stand with your feet together and place your right hand on your hip to help you keep your upper body straight.

COUNTS: Every swing takes one count.

STEP 1: Gently swing your right leg out to the front. Then swing it back as though it was a pendulum. Lift your leg no higher than six inches off the floor. Do eight Leg Pendulums on this side.

STEP 2: Move the chair to your right and switch hands. Do eight Leg Pendulums with your left leg.

POINTERS:

◆ Keep your hips facing forward.

◆ Your upper body should not move.

◆ Tuck your buttocks and lower abdomen slightly forward.

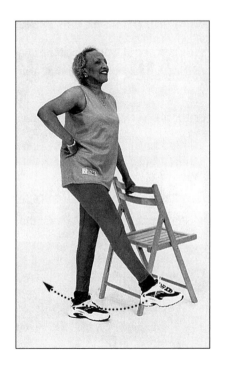

DANCE ROUTINE

*"I thought I just had to live with the pain, but there is hope.
The dancing is fun and gentle. I feel good again."*
—PAIGE, THIRTY-NINE

It is time to put on your favorite music and let yourself go. Together, music and dance promote the return of good health. Use the dance routine to forget your troubles, release your tension, and move beyond the pain.

MUSICAL SUGGESTION: Lou Vega, "Mambo Number 5."

STARTING POSITION: Stand in the center of the room with your arms by your sides.

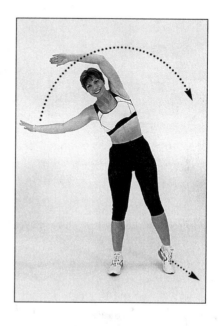

THE SHOWGIRL STRUT: Step to the right, swinging your arms from left to right overhead like a Las Vegas showgirl with attitude. Then touch your left foot to the side. Step to the left, swinging your arms overhead from right to left. Then touch your right foot to the side.

Do eight sets.

Then come to a stationary position. Place your hands on your hips in preparation for Reach for the Stars.

REACH FOR THE STARS: Reach your right arm up, as though you are trying to touch a star. Then reach farther for a second count. Lower your right hand to your hip on two counts.

Now reach up the same way with your left arm.

Do four sets.

Relax your arms to your sides and move on to Wash the Windows.

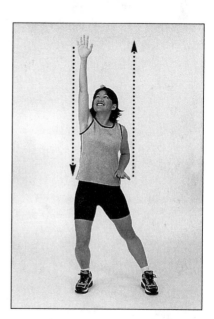

WASH THE WINDOWS: Make four large circles in front of your body with your right arm, as though you are washing a giant window. Let your hips rock from side to side with the same momentum. Relax your right arm.

Make four circles with your left arm. Relax your left arm.

Continue immediately with Step-Touch.

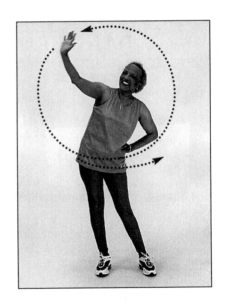

STEP-TOUCH: Step to the right, swinging your arms up and to the right. Then touch your left foot to the side and clap your hands at the same time. Step to the left, swinging your arms up and to the left. Touch your right foot to the side and clap your hands at the same time.

Do four sets.

Go through the whole Dance Routine four times, unless you feel too tired or achy, in which case feel free to stop. Then take a slow walk around the room for one minute, or walk in place, to lower your heart rate. Breathe deeply in and out to feed your body oxygen. Make sure you drink some water.

Spend a few quiet minutes doing the Healing Visualization that follows.

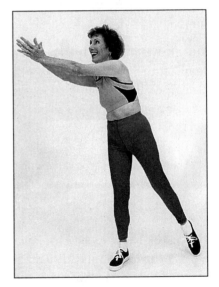

HEALING VISUALIZATION
FOR PAIN

Sit down in a chair and make yourself comfortable. Close your eyes and check in with how your body feels. Scan your feet, ankles, and legs, then your hands, wrists, and arms. Allow them to relax. Let your belly release. Scan your back, chest, shoulders, neck, and head. Let your jaw and the muscles on the front of your face relax. Identify any places of pain and tightness in your body without changing anything.

Take long, deep breaths in through your nose and out through your mouth. On every in-breath, visualize a green-tinged golden light filling your body. This light is healing. On every out-breath, release dark clouds of pain, emotion, and tension.

Now imagine a burning hot, bright orange-red sun. The sun surrounds and embraces your pain. See your pain as an ice cube being placed on that sun and melting. As the ice melts it changes into cool and refreshing water.

Say three times, "My pain is melting away." Allow that to mean whatever it means to you.

Spend a few moments in silence and then, when you feel ready, open your eyes.

COMBATING FATIGUE

"Cancer is an obnoxious disease and makes the body do

obnoxious things, so keep your sense of humor."

—*Twin, fifty-eight*

*L*ike pain, fatigue is a major quality-of-life issue for survivors. It can

get in the way of earning a living and make it hard to socialize with your fam-

ily and friends. When your energy level is low, you can even have trouble

climbing stairs or concentrating on ordinary tasks like housecleaning. You

may lose your desire for sexual intimacy. Fatigue can result from surgery and

anesthesia, chemotherapy and radiation, weight gain or depression—and can

last an extremely long time. Being kind to your body and self-nurturing is the

way to live with fatigue. As unwelcome and frustrating as fatigue may be, the needs of your body cannot be ignored or resisted.

Twin is a five-year survivor of breast cancer. She had fatigue from the onset of her treatment, and even now on some days she feels as if she is walking on stumps not legs. A lumpectomy with a node dissection was followed by fourteen weeks of chemotherapy that made her incredibly weak and sick. Then she underwent radiation treatment. The radiation exhausted and burned her so much that she thought she was falling apart. These days she often feels worn out. Sometimes she can go for a week or ten days without feeling tired, and then suddenly she gets fatigued to the point where she just has to go to bed.

To combat her fatigue, Twin is careful about what she eats and about getting enough rest. She drinks fresh juices, takes herbal supplements, and attends Focus on Healing classes. She has found that when she pushes herself to come to an afternoon class despite her exhaustion, she leaves feeling rejuvenated. Exercise gives her energy and motivation that last her through the remainder of the evening.

Exercise and rest, especially getting enough sleep, can make a tremendous difference in your energy reserves and how well you are able to cope with whatever is on your plate. Exercise can help you release toxins, build up your endorphin levels, elevate your mood, and restore some of the muscle tone that can be lost after even a few days recuperating from surgery. In addition, when fatigue lingers, you would do well to seek the advice of your physician. Have your doctor check your hemoglobin levels. The mild anemia associated with treatment can be corrected in many cases.

FATIGUE SPECIFICS FOR SURVIVORS The "Combating Fatigue" routine can help raise your energy so long as you take it easy. Overexertion would defeat the purpose, so you want to work just hard enough to release endorphins—natural painkillers—and oxygen into your bloodstream. If you stop before you feel overly taxed or tired, you will find that you end up with more energy, not more fatigue. So throughout the routine, be conscious of your energy level. If you start to feel more exhausted than when you started, that is your signal to rest. You've done enough.

THE COMBATING FATIGUE ROUTINE
- The Basic Warm-up (pp. 15–23)
- Single-Arm Reach
- Overhead Side Stretch
- The Crawl
- The Backstroke
- The Breaststroke
- Single and Double Leg Lifts
- Seated March
- Heel Lifts
- Foot Flex
- Seated Dance Routine
- Healing Visualization

SINGLE-ARM REACH

Begin here, after doing the Basic Warm-up. The feeling of the Single-Arm Reach is as though someone is pulling your arm and saying "Come with me!" and you are responding "No, I don't want to go!" and pulling back. Resistance is what makes the stretch happen. You should feel it in your shoulder blades and across your rib cage.

STARTING POSITION: Stand with your feet hip-width apart. Your left hand is on your hip.

STEP 1: Raise your right arm to shoulder height. Then move it to the left across your chest as far as possible. Keep your arm straight and pull back with your right shoulder. Your right hand should remain in place, resisting your shoulder, so you get a good stretch. Relax your arms by your sides.

Do four stretches with your right arm.

STEP 2: Now put your right hand on your hip and repeat the stretch four times with your left arm. Relax your arms by your sides.

POINTERS:

◆ Keep your arms straight.

◆ Keep your hips facing front.

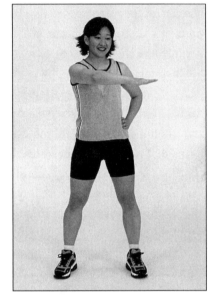

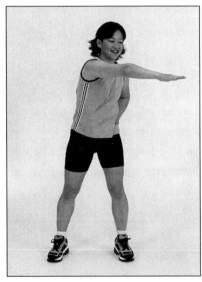

OVERHEAD SIDE STRETCH

This exercise can give you a surge of energy. Stretching the muscles and scar tissue along your rib cage helps open up your breathing apparatus. Oxygen relieves fatigue.

STARTING POSITION: Stand with your feet hip-width apart; your arms hanging at your sides with the palms facing inward.

STEP 1: Swing your right arm slowly out to the side and up over your head. Your palm should be facing out. Gently tilt your body to the left and reach to the left with your right arm. Hold this position for two deep breaths in and out.

STEP 2: Return your body to an upright position and bring your right arm back down, making a slow, reaching arc.

Repeat the stretch on your left side.

Do two more stretches on each side.

POINTERS:

◆ Keep your palm facing outward even at the height of the stretch.

◆ Be gentle and move slowly.

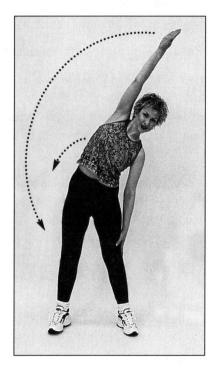

THE CRAWL

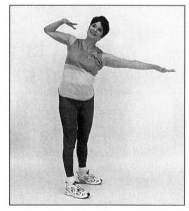

The Crawl is a soothing way of exercising. Much like actual swimming, it is gentle and helps build energy. I told my class once, "Imagine that you're Esther Williams." When they replied, "Who's that?" I knew that my classes were getting younger and I was getting older.

STARTING POSITION: Stand with your feet hip-width apart. Your arms should be straight out in front of your body at shoulder height—or as high as you can lift them.

COUNTS: Every arm circle takes eight counts.

STEP 1: To do the Crawl, your arms must cycle independently. Lower your right arm down to your side, then bend your right elbow and bring the arm up to shoulder height. From shoulder height, continue the movement by extending the arm straight up in the air.

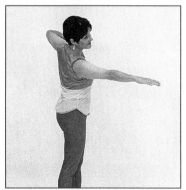

STEP 2: At the same time, bring your left arm down to your side, then bend the left elbow and bring your left arm up to shoulder height. As the left arm is rising, circle the right arm forward and down to the starting position. As the left arm continues straight up into the air, lower your right arm to your side.

Circle both arms four times. Turn your head to the right as your right hand reaches your shoulder and then turn it to the left as your left hand reaches your shoulder. Try to find a steady rhythm.

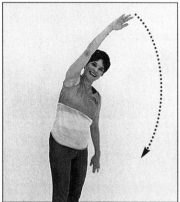

POINTERS:

◆ Always turn your head toward the arm that is at your shoulder.

◆ Your movements are continuous and flowing.

◆ Imagine the resistance of the water.

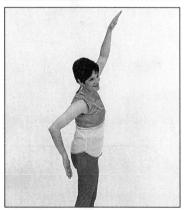

THE BACKSTROKE

This exercise helps you to increase your range of motion—you feel less tired when you are more flexible since you no longer have to exert as much energy on the effort of simple movements.

STARTING POSITION: Stand with your feet hip-width apart. Place your arms straight in front of your body at shoulder height.

COUNTS: Each arm circle takes four counts.

STEP 1: Keeping your right arm as straight as possible, circle it back and down, and then return it to the starting position.

STEP 2: As your right arm is on its way down, begin making a similar backward circle with your left arm.

Make four circles with each arm.

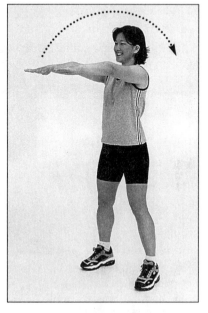

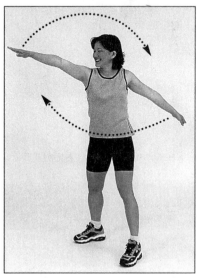

THE BREASTSTROKE

The Breaststroke increases your stamina. Stronger arm muscles are more efficient and require less energy to move.

STARTING POSITION: Stand with your feet hip-width apart and your knees slightly bent. Bring your hands together in front of your chest at shoulder height and let your elbows come up and out to the side. Your palms are facing front. Lean forward a tiny bit and look straight ahead.

COUNTS: Every Breaststroke takes four counts, or one count for each movement.

STEP 1: Push your palms forward, keeping them at shoulder height.

STEP 2: When your arms are fully extended in front of you, circle them out to your sides and simultaneously straighten your legs.

STEP 3: Keeping your legs straight, drop your arms to your sides. Then bend your knees and return to the starting position.
   Repeat four times.

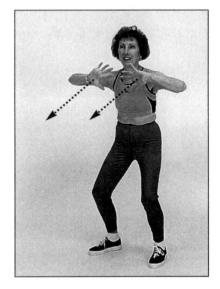

POINTERS:

◆ Be sure to spread your arms wide to the side to feel the expanse of the stretch across your chest.

◆ This is a great exercise for breathing. Inhale as you move your arms forward and exhale as you return them to the starting position.

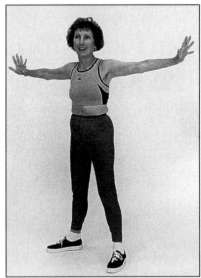

SINGLE AND DOUBLE LEG LIFTS

You need to get a full body workout if you want to increase your energy and strength. This exercise begins to work the lower body.

WHAT YOU NEED FOR THIS EXERCISE: A chair.

STARTING POSITION: Sit all the way back in your chair, but remain upright instead of leaning back. Your feet should be flat on the floor, your spine straight, and your shoulders lightly pressed down. Think about pulling your tummy in, while you keep breathing.

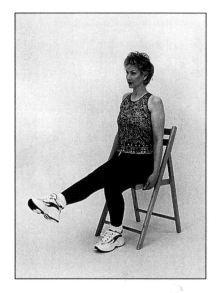

COUNTS: Every movement takes two counts.

STEP 1: Straighten your right leg in front of you and point your toes. Hold for two counts. Then lower it to the starting position and relax your foot. Do eight Single Leg Lifts.
   Repeat with your left leg.

STEP 2: Next, straighten both legs in front of you, pointing the toes. Hold for two counts. As you lower your legs to the starting position relax your feet. Do four Double Leg Lifts.

POINTERS:

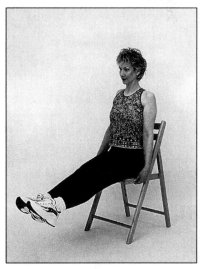

◆ For extra stability you may hold on to the edges of your chair. Use your arms to give you some leverage as you lift your legs.

◆ Concentrating on your quadriceps, the muscles located on the front of your thighs, can help you reap the benefits of this simple exercise, which uses several muscle groups.

◆ Holding your stomach in will help you remain upright.

◆ Move slowly through the repetitions. It's a simple exercise but it has many benefits.

SEATED MARCH

"This program has given me confidence. I have made great progress in relieving my fatigue and stress, and I feel in control again."

—JANE, FORTY-TWO

Remember, fatigue involves the whole body. Marching works and strengthens your leg muscles. Imagine that you are in a parade and have fun.

WHAT YOU NEED FOR THIS EXERCISE: A chair.

STARTING POSITION: Sit on the edge of your chair with a straight back. Feel free to swing your arms during the marches to get your blood pumping. Alternatively, you may hold on to the edges of your chair for stability.

COUNTS: March for sixteen counts.

STEP 1: March your legs, first right and then left, eight times.

POINTER:

◆ Stop if you get tired.

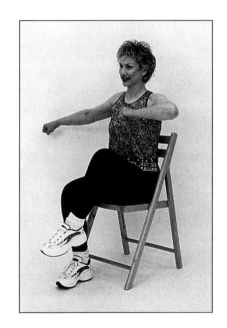

HEEL LIFTS

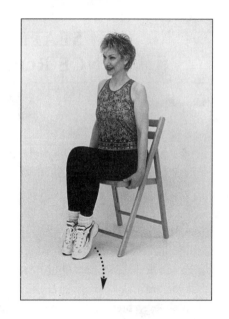

This exercise is easy to do and it builds strength in your lower legs. Remember, there is no pressure in this program, no guilt if you have to stop and rest—just take your time and work slower if you need to.

WHAT YOU NEED FOR THIS EXERCISE: A chair.

STARTING POSITION: Sit on the edge of your chair. Your hands are either clasping the edges of the chair for stability or resting in your lap.

COUNTS: Each Heel Lift takes four counts.

STEP 1: Slowly lift your heels so you are resting on the balls of your feet. Then lower them down again. Repeat four times.

FOOT FLEX

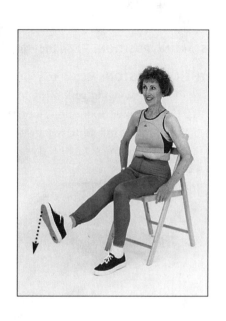

The Foot Flex helps build strength in your feet and ankles, which are important in holding your body upright.

WHAT YOU NEED FOR THIS EXERCISE: a chair.

STARTING POSITION: Sit back in your chair with your feet flat on the floor, your spine erect, your shoulders down and back, and your tummy lifted.

COUNTS: Each flex or point takes one count.

STEP 1: Straighten your right leg so that it's parallel to the floor. In this position, first flex your foot, and then point your foot. Flex and point your right foot four times. Then lower your leg.
   Repeat with your left leg and foot.

STEP 2: Now straighten both legs and point and flex both feet eight times.

SEATED
DANCE ROUTINE

"I feel younger and more alive after doing this program—and have much more energy."

—NAOMI, FIFTY-NINE

Doing the entire routine for fatigue is a goal. I know it's a lot to accomplish. Please don't feel disappointed if you can't do everything today. Instead, hold your head high and smile, and know that you are making progress! Keep in mind that it's okay for you to stop—even preferable—when you have reached your limit.

I have designed this as a seated routine to accommodate your fatigue. But if you're feeling energetic and the exercises you have done so far in this chapter haven't worn you out, you may substitute a standing dance routine from another chapter. The routine in "Exploring Your Femininity" may be a good level to try next.

WHAT YOU NEED FOR THE SEATED DANCE ROUTINE: A chair.

MUSICAL SUGGESTION: Cherry Poppin' Daddies, "Zoot Suit Riot."

STARTING POSITION: Sit on the edge of your chair.

THE CHARLESTON: Step onto your left foot and kick your right leg forward, swinging your arms to the right as you kick. Then step backward with your right foot, touch your left foot behind you, and at the same time swing your arms to the left.

Repeat four times.

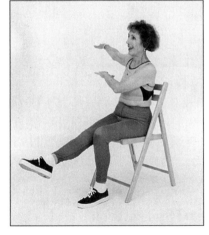

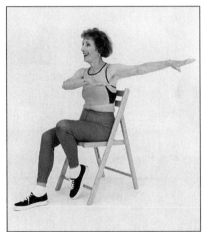

KNEE BOUNCE: Put your hands on your knees and bounce your knees in and out on a count of two. When your knees touch, switch your hands to rest on the opposite knees. When they touch again put them back on the same knee.

Bounce in and out four times.

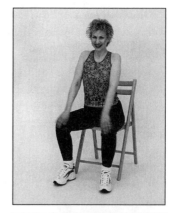

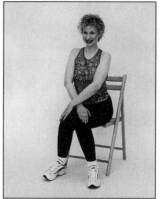

TOE-HEEL WALK: Now you're going to walk your feet to the right, moving your heels and then toes four times. Then reverse direction and walk your feet back to center, moving your heels and then toes four times. Hold on to your chair for balance.

Repeat moving to the left side.

Do four sets.

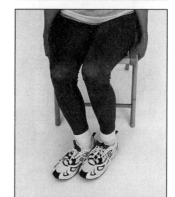

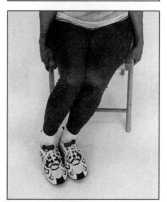

THE WINDSHIELD WIPER: Now bring your hands up to your shoulders with your palms facing forward. Wipe your hands right and then left eight times.

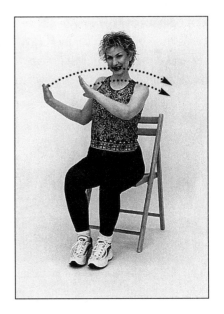

Do the whole routine over from the beginning as many times as possible until the song ends. Please remember not to overexert yourself. Have a drink of water and rest for a few minutes.

POINTERS:

◆ Smile and have fun.

◆ Just move. It doesn't matter whether you're doing it exactly "right."

HEALING VISUALIZATION
FOR FATIGUE

Sit comfortably in a chair and close your eyes. Get in touch with all the parts of your body, from your feet and legs, to your arms and shoulders, stomach, chest, and back, up to the crown of your head. Feel a rooted connection to the center of the earth and as if your head is open to the sky. You are present here and now. There is no longer anything to fight against. Let go of any tension in your jaw, throat, and hips.

Inhale deeply. With every in-breath, imagine that your spine is being filled with a powerful red light. The color red rises up through your tailbone like a thermometer rising and moves past your heart and enters your brain. As you exhale, let go of all your resistance to fatigue.

Now imagine yourself standing up and walking out of the room you're in. You go down to a phone booth where you rip off your clothes. Surprise! Underneath you're wearing tights and a cape. There's a big T sewn on your chest (for "Thriver"). You can feel energy pulsing through your body like electricity. You run out into the street and leap up and fly over a tall building. You can do anything!

Say three times: "I am filled with energy. I am filled with life. I have the power to do it all."

When you're done flying, open your eyes.

EMOTIONAL RECOVERY

*"After the program I was so proud of myself. I had a wonderful feeling
that my life wasn't hopeless anymore."*

—*Gerri, sixty-one*

Anger is one of the primary emotions that survivors often experience. It is a natural response to trauma. You may be angry at your body for betraying you, angry with your doctors for cutting you, angry with the people around you, and angry with God for your suffering. Another common emotion is grief. You may feel grief over the loss of your breast, grief at having your life interrupted, and grief at the uncertainty of your future. I know how you feel, because I've felt those things, too. Cancer recovery can be an emotional journey.

When Gerri retired after thirty years as a teacher, she dreamed of pursuing her passion for amateur ballroom dancing. Her favorite dances were the tango, foxtrot, and quickstep waltz. Then she was diagnosed with cancer in both breasts and had to undergo surgery. The resulting physical losses hit her hard. Radiation treatments left Gerri with a chronic heart arrhythmia, unable to walk twenty steps without stopping to catch her breath. Depression set in as she realized that her plans for dancing through the rest of her life had evaporated.

A year later Gerri joined a Focus on Healing class to expand her range of motion. In the process, she discovered that being around other women who could relate to her story made her feel less isolated. She also learned that she could lend emotional support to others. When one survivor in her class was worried about an impending hair loss, Gerri had no qualms about pulling off her wig to demonstrate how easy it is to hide. No one in the class had known she was wearing a wig. Listening to music, participating in movement, and enjoying the company of friends lifted her spirits and restored her sense of wholeness.

Karen had initially slipped through the cracks of modern medicine. At twenty-six she felt a lump in her breast but her doctor reassured her that it was nothing, saying, "You're too young." So she had believed she was a hypochondriac, until six years later a biopsy proved that she had an aggressive cancer. After her treatment, which included surgery, chemotherapy, and radiation, the formerly active aerobics instructor sank into a deep depression and became a self-described couch potato. She no longer wanted to do anything but mope around feeling sorry for herself.

Even the birth of her third child a year after treatment couldn't resolve this deep sadness. The only people who knew what was going on with her emotionally were her immediate family.

Karen was finally directed to a Focus on Healing class. Her chest wall was still tender to the touch and she had guarded it, the pain seeming to grow with each passing year. But she learned that when she did the exercises, they relieved some of her pain and she felt less emotionally guarded. As she got stronger, she found herself smiling and laughing again and remembered how much she had always loved to be active. The whole experience was so emotionally healing, in fact, that at age thirty-eight she made the twin decisions to go to nursing school and become a certified Focus on Healing instructor. She wanted to offer the gift of the program to other survivors struggling with their own issues. Today her direction is clear, her mind is clear, her depression is gone, and she is thriving.

Many survivors become depressed and stay that way for a long time. A study done at the University of Michigan found that as many as 64 percent of breast cancer survivors are still depressed ten years after surgery. However, it also showed that survivors who get regular exercise feel less depressed and anxious than more sedentary ones. Working up a sweat gives them an endorphin rush, circulating natural painkilling chemicals that act like opiates through the bloodstream. It also makes them feel more in control of their lives and thus better able to handle stress. Unwanted stress chemicals like adrenaline can be eliminated from the body through perspiration. The study found that these results could be achieved by lightly exercising for thirty minutes four times a week.

Let's face it, as survivors we feel many different emotions. As relieved as we are to be alive, we may also fear many aspects of having cancer, including the diagnosis, surgery, radiation, chemotherapy, lymphedema, recurrence, weight gain, and other losses in our lives. Many of us go through a period in which we experience a lack of self-esteem or confidence in our ability to meet new challenges. This is a lot to endure on top of everything else. Exercise can help us tremendously. It boosts our resilience, it's fun, and it brings joy back into our lives.

EMOTIONAL RECOVERY SPECIFICS FOR SURVIVORS You should practice this routine whenever you want to release strong emotions. All of the exercises include spoken words that should be said with as much emphasis as you can muster. Instead of resisting your emotions, you should acknowledge and embrace them and let them go.

After the physical work, there are two different forms of relaxation and meditation exercises that you can practice to get in touch with and explore your inner feelings. Regular contemplation and relaxation have been proven to soothe the nervous system, and stabilize mood swings and overpowering emotions. Please experiment and use whichever makes you feel better.

THE EMOTIONAL RECOVERY ROUTINE

- ◆ The Basic Warm-up (pp. 15–23)
- ◆ Leg Pendulums
- ◆ Toe Taps
- ◆ Single-Arm Reach
- ◆ Reach for the Stars
- ◆ Hold the Walls Back
- ◆ Hold Up the Ceiling
- ◆ Wash the Windows
- ◆ Scrub a Spot
- ◆ Side Arm Swings
- ◆ Lower Body Ultimates (pp. 169–174)
- ◆ Dance Routine
- ◆ Progressive Relaxation
- ◆ Meditation on the Breath

LEG PENDULUMS

You can use Leg Pendulums to release negative emotions, such as anger and frustration. Think of something that really ticks you off or an emotion that has been weighing on you, and then use the force of that emotion to swing your leg. As you move, repeat out loud, "Get rid of it!" As you swing, imagine the negative feelings being released from your body.

WHAT YOU NEED FOR THIS EXERCISE: A supporting chair.

STARTING POSITION: Place the chair to your left and hold on to it with your left hand. Stand with your feet together and place your right hand on your hip to help you keep your upper body straight.

COUNTS: Every swing takes one count.

STEP 1: Gently swing your right leg out to the front. Then swing it back as though it was a pendulum. Lift your leg no higher than six inches off the floor. Do eight Leg Pendulums on this side.

STEP 2: Move the chair to your right and switch hands. Do eight Leg Pendulums with your left leg.

POINTERS:

◆ Keep your hips facing forward.

◆ Your upper body should not move.

◆ Tuck your buttocks and lower abdomen slightly forward.

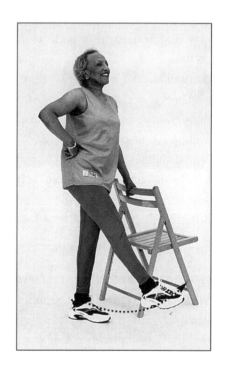

TOE TAPS

There are many challenging aspects to surviving breast cancer. One of these is feeling out of control. Another is being told to do what you don't want to do or feel capable of doing—even when it's for your own good. Toe Taps are an opportunity to assert your voice and put your foot down. With every tap, firmly repeat out loud, "No!" and let yourself really mean it.

STARTING POSITION: Stand with your feet together. Your arms are raised out to the sides at shoulder height. Use a supporting

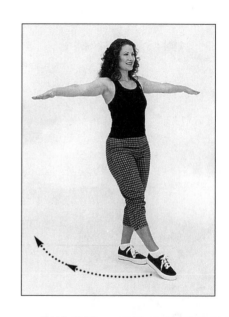

chair if you have concerns about your balance, placing it on your left side when you are working your right leg and vice versa.

COUNTS: Every Toe Tap takes one count.

STEP 1: Tap your right foot to the front. Tap it to the side. Tap it behind you. Then bring your feet together.

STEP 2: Repeat with your left foot.
   Do two sets.

SINGLE-ARM REACH

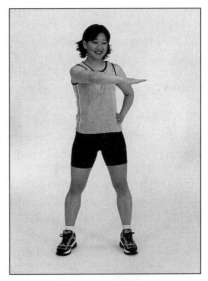

Some days you may want to try new things. Other days you may want to collapse and be left alone. Use the Single-Arm Reach to practice making those choices—to see what it feels like to be both active and passive. As you stretch your arm, say, "Yes!" and when you release, say, "No."

STARTING POSITION: Stand with your feet hip-width apart. Your left hand is on your hip.

STEP 1: Raise your right arm to shoulder height. Then move it to the left across your chest as far as possible. Keep your right arm straight. Reach your right arm farther to the left as though someone were pulling on it. Resist with your right shoulder, as if you were pulling back. Then release the tension.
   Do four stretches with your right arm.

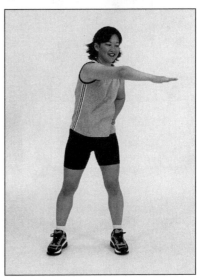

STEP 2: Reverse your arms. Repeat the stretch four times with your left arm.

POINTERS:
◆ Keep your arms straight.
◆ Keep your hips facing front.

REACH FOR THE STARS

This is a chance for some positive words of encouragement—a confidence builder. Among other things, you can be proud of participating in this program and focusing on your health and well-being. Imagine a goal or a dream that you care deeply about, put it up on the ceiling, and reach for it, saying, "I can do it! I can do it!"

STARTING POSITION: Stand with your feet hip-width apart. Your hands are on your hips.

COUNTS: Every reach takes four counts.

STEP 1: Reach your right arm up, as though you are trying to touch a star. Then reach farther for a second count. Lower your right hand to your hip on two counts.

STEP 2: Now reach up the same way with your left arm.
    Do four sets.

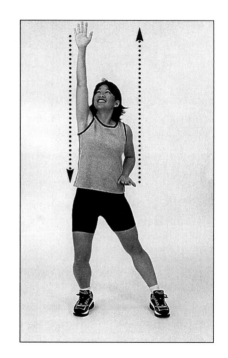

HOLD THE WALLS BACK

Breast cancer is a frightening adversary. When I was diagnosed I felt as though I was under attack from almost every side. Now, after five years, I still get nervous when I go for my routine check-ups. This exercise enables you to take any feelings of being overwhelmed and channel them into physical energy. Command the world, "Stay back!"

STARTING POSITION: Stand with your right foot forward and your knees straight. Your hands are at your shoulder, palms facing forward.

COUNTS: Four counts to straighten and four counts to bend.

STEP 1: As you slowly bend your legs, gently push your palms forward until your arms are straight—as though you are pushing against a wall. Keep your wrists flexed.

STEP 2: Now slowly straighten your knees and return your hands to the starting position.

Switch your legs so that your left leg is forward and repeat.

POINTER:

◆ If you have difficulty maintaining your balance, you may do this with your feet together.

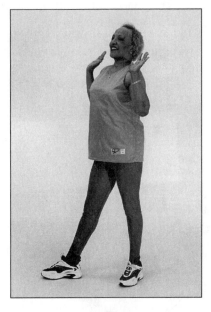

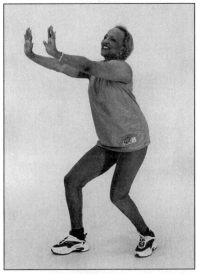

HOLD UP THE CEILING

Feeling stressed? Mad as heck? Say, "Get that stress off me!" as you do this movement.

STARTING POSITION: Stand with your feet slightly apart and your knees bent. Your hands are at your shoulders with your palms flexed toward the ceiling.

COUNTS: Four counts to straighten and four counts to bend.

STEP 1: Gently push your arms up toward the ceiling as you straighten your knees. Hold. Bend your knees and return your hands to your shoulders.

Repeat four times.

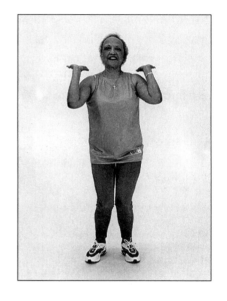

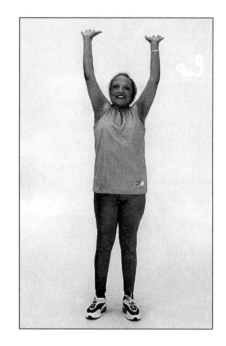

WASH THE WINDOWS

Are you starting to feel better? Why not celebrate? Enjoy your lighter side by repeating, "I feel good."

STARTING POSITION: Stand with your feet hip-width apart and your knees slightly bent.

COUNTS: Every circle takes four counts.

STEP 1: Make four large circles in front of your body with your right arm, as though you are washing a giant window. Let your hips rock freely from side to side.

Now make four large circles with your left arm.

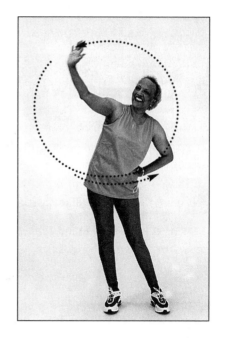

SCRUB A SPOT

Think of a nuisance or frustration in your life right now that you'd like to let go of. As you do this exercise, repeat out loud, "I release this."

STARTING POSITION: Stand with your feet hip-width apart and your knees slightly bent. Your right arm is extended in front of you at chest height, wrist flexed and palm facing outward.

COUNTS: Scrub for eight counts with each hand.

STEP 1: Make rapid, tiny circles with your right hand as if you were scrubbing an incorrigible spot off a pot.

STEP 2: Switch arms and repeat with your left hand.

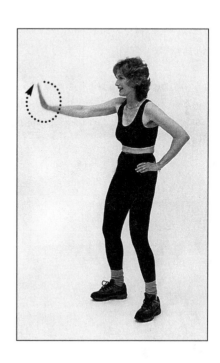

SIDE ARM SWINGS

By this point, you've probably been on an emotional roller coaster. Hopefully your load is a little lighter and life seems brighter. You can use this exercise to draw upon your passion for living. As you swing your arms, affirm that positive spirit by repeating, "I feel great. I feel free. I feel ready."

STARTING POSITION: Stand with your feet hip-width apart and your arms hanging at your sides.

COUNTS: Every swing takes two counts.

STEP 1: Swing both arms easily and freely to the right. As you swing your arms, shift your weight onto your right foot and allow your left heel to lift off the floor. Follow your hands with your head.

STEP 2: Now swing your arms back down and then up to the left, shifting your weight to your left foot and allowing your right heel to lift off the floor. Follow your hands with your head.

Do eight sets.

At this point in the Emotional Recovery program, you should add on the Lower Body Ultimates (pp. 169–174). After you complete those exercises, continue with the dance routine on the next page.

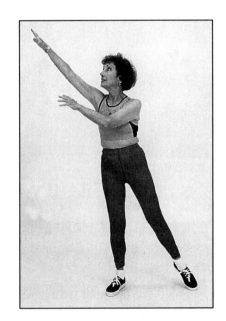

DANCE ROUTINE

Your emotional journey continues with this playful dance routine. Set aside your daily stresses and plans and let yourself go. You deserve this time to move and be free. Life does not have to be a downer.

MUSICAL SUGGESTION: Carlos Santana, "Africa Bamba."

STARTING POSITION: Stand with your feet hip-width apart and your knees slightly bent. Your arms hang by your sides.

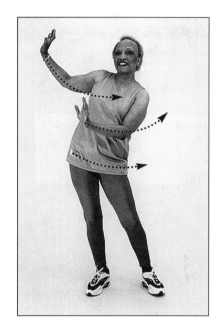

HIP SWING: Swing your hips slowly from right to left and back again eight times. Allow your arms to move naturally from side to side; there's no specific arm motion you must follow.

STEP-TOUCH FORWARD AND BACK: Step forward with the right foot. Then touch your left to your right foot while clapping your hands. Now step back onto your left foot and touch your right foot to your left foot while clapping your hands.

Do four sets. Bend your elbows and raise your hands to your shoulders in preparation for Step-Together-Step-Touch.

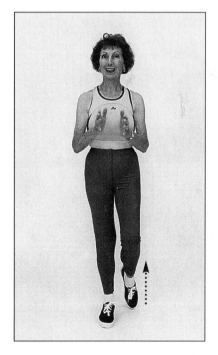

STEP-TOGETHER-STEP-TOUCH: You're going to travel right. Step out and shift your weight onto your right foot and step your left foot beside it. Step out again onto your right foot. This time touch your left foot beside the right without placing your weight on it. As you touch, push your hands straight up over your head, wrists flexed palms up.

Bring your hands back to shoulder height as you begin to travel left, stepping out with your left foot. Do the same series in reverse: step-together-step-touch. Push your hands to the ceiling as you touch your right foot.

Do four sets. Let your arms drop down to your sides again.

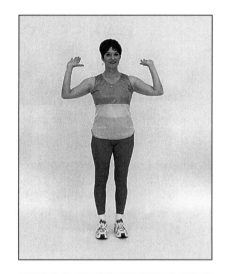

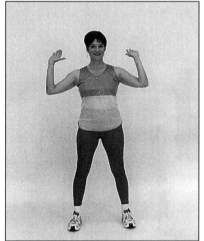

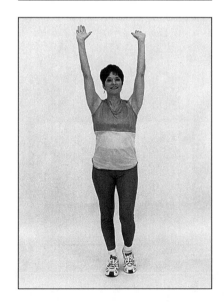

TRAVELING TAP STEP: Smack the ball of your right foot a little in front of you, as if there's a tap on the bottom of your shoe. Then put your right heel down. Do the same tap step on the left so that you begin to travel forward. Swing your arms from side to side as you step.

Do four sets. Lift your arms overhead in preparation for the Showgirl Strut.

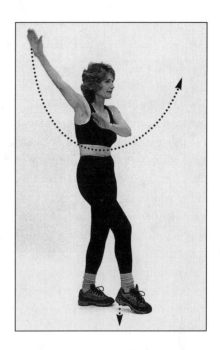

THE SHOWGIRL STRUT: Step to the right, swinging your arms from left to right overhead like a Las Vegas showgirl with attitude. Then touch your left foot to the side. Step to the left, swinging your arms overhead from right to left. Then touch your right foot to the side.

Do eight sets.

Repeat the whole routine as many times as you can until your song ends. Then walk leisurely around the room to slow your heart rate. Have a refreshing drink of water.

Now, for relaxation, try one or both of the exercises that follow.

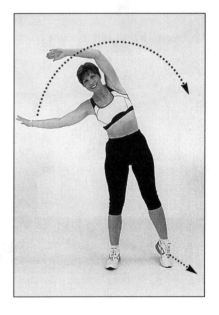

PROGRESSIVE RELAXATION

The purpose of this relaxation technique is to create mental and emotional stillness through physical stillness. When you are lying down, you don't have to do anything. You are completely supported by a bed, a couch, the floor, or the earth. Gravity helps you to sink, your muscles release, and you can venture into a state of pure being. It is a process of letting go. It is a time for silence and nondoing.

I recommend that you give yourself permission to relax for fifteen to forty-five minutes. Find a quiet place to lie down where you won't be disturbed. Turn off the telephone, ask your family to respect your privacy—lock the door if need be. You may find yourself falling asleep in the process, and that's okay, you probably need the rest. Or you may drift from thought to thought, and that's okay, too. There is no right or wrong way to do this exercise. It is the absence of doing that you are seeking.

Lie on your back and close your eyes. Remind yourself, "Do less." Notice what that feels like for a few moments: doing less.

Starting with your right foot, tense all the muscles in your toes. Really scrunch them up, good and tight. Next, add tension to your foot—the ball, the arch, the heel, and the ankle. Keep moving up your leg, part by part, doing the same thing. Tense your calf muscles. Tense your knees, then your thighs. Let your whole leg lift slightly off the floor. Then release everything completely. Drop your leg. Let all that tension go.

Now move your attention to your left leg and repeat the same process of tensing and releasing.

Next, squeeze your buttocks as hard as you can. Tense your hip muscles. Tense your lower abdomen. Hold on until the intensity is almost too much to bear, then release. Let it all go.

Now begin with your right hand. Make a fist, tighten your forearm, tighten your biceps and triceps and your right shoulder. Let them lift off the floor. When you cannot tighten anymore, let it drop. Release completely.

Move to your left arm and repeat the same process of tensing and letting go.

Then tighten and release your stomach muscles and chest. Move to your back. When you have let those go, clench your shoulders up to your ears. Hold for a few moments, and then let them go. Tense and release your neck.

Finally, contract all the muscles in your face. Purse your lips and cheeks. Squeeze your eyelids and nose. Even tighten your scalp. Then do the opposite. Open your eyes and mouth and stretch them as wide as you can. Let that all go.

Close your eyes again and notice how you feel. Remain still and remind yourself again, "Do less." Run a quick scan through all those body parts and feel them released.

Sink into relaxation. Stay there as long as you like and drift.

Be with yourself.

MEDITATION ON THE BREATH

Meditation is much simpler than many people realize. There are all kinds of formal traditions and styles of meditation, such as observing the flame of a candle, walking in a circle, or holding various postures, and you may wish to explore some of these. These are means of transcending activity and getting in touch with your core self. Your core is the part of you that simply is, and was, and will be. Not your body, not your thoughts, not even your emotions. There is a tremendous power at your core because it is neutral.

Meditation differs from visualization because you are not purposefully playing with the images in your mind. Rather, the aim is to still your thoughts, or perhaps find your way into the gap between thoughts. When images or ideas do come up, which is almost inevitable, you should let them flow through your mind without attaching to them. In this particular meditation, you will keep your focus on your breath as an anchor to assist you in this purpose.

There is no right or wrong amount of time to meditate. I would suggest setting aside a minimum of fifteen minutes at first, and then to experiment with your own preferences. There is also no right or wrong time of day to meditate. The right time is when you do it.

Sit quietly in a comfortable position. Ground and stabilize your feet. Place your hands in a stable position in your lap. Make sure your spine is supported and erect. Your head is level or tipped slightly forward. Your shoulders are released. Close your eyes. Hold this position for the duration of the meditation. The instructions are simple: Breathe in and out through your nose. Without changing anything, observe your sensations. Follow each single breath as it travels through your nostrils, down your throat, and expands your chest and belly. Follow the flow of the breath back up and out.

When your mind wanders, gently turn your attention back to the breath. Allow your experience to be whatever it is.

The more you practice meditation, the more benefits you reap. The more you can tap into your core observer self, the more neutral you are as events swirl around you, the more accepting you can become, and the better able you are to face any challenges that lay ahead.

LIVING WITH LYMPHEDEMA

"The exercises are wonderful. Even though I am wearing a glove and sleeve,
my movements seem to be getting better and I feel stronger."

—*Janet, sixty-four*

*I*f you have had a lumpectomy, simple mastectomy, modified radical mastectomy, or axillary node dissection, often combined with radiation, you may be at risk for developing lymphedema. Lymphedema is a persistent and often debilitating swelling caused by a profusion of lymph. Lymph is a colorless fluid formed in the tissue spaces throughout the body. It normally passes through the lymph nodes, which perform many functions, including purifying the lymph of harmful bacteria and viruses—a process vital to wound healing—and producing infection-fighting cells and substances. The lymphatic system plays a crucial role in the immune system.

It is common to have a few or many lymph nodes removed during breast surgery in order to diagnose the spread of cancer and plan your treatment. As a result of node removal, the lymphatic system becomes impaired and an abnormal amount of protein-rich lymph fluid collects in the tissue of the affected arm. Sometimes gentle exercise will improve the swelling. But a woman with lymphedema should make sure never to overtire her arm.

Phyllis is a two-year survivor of breast cancer, and lymphedema has been a persistent issue for her from early on. Only four months after her chemotherapy ended, she noticed some pain in her surgical arm one evening. By the next morning when she woke up, her arm and shoulder hurt much more severely and looked red, and she found herself running a high temperature. Her doctor examined her and diagnosed her with lymphedema and a severe bacterial infection. She checked into the hospital for a week until her fever and other symptoms could be brought under control.

Phyllis found out about the Focus on Healing program from a social worker at the hospital. She also joined a lymphedema support group and learned how to do self-manual lymphatic drainage and to bandage her arm properly. In addition, her physical therapist fitted her with a sleeve to wear while she goes about her daily activities. Through all of these steps she has kept her lymphedema under control for more than a year. She occasionally experiences discomfort when she vacuums or does yard work, and has found that just reaching into a high cabinet can sometimes trigger swelling. But she knows the exercises will help keep her swelling down. She even does them in the shower when she is short of time. Maintaining circulation in her arm is the key. She has made a lifelong commitment to the program.

If you receive a diagnosis of lymphedema, you will be given a compression sleeve or wrapping to wear on the affected arm. This must be worn every time you exercise. It is likely that you will also be referred to a certified lymphedema specialist—this can be a physical therapist, an occupational therapist, or a massage therapist who is trained in complete decongestive therapy. Your therapist helps you treat your condition and teaches you and your loved ones to manage it through exercise, diet, self-manual lymphatic drainage, and bandaging. You can contact the National Lymphedema Network for more information (see Resources).

LYMPHEDEMA SPECIFICS FOR SURVIVORS The "Living with Lymphedema" routine is designed to maintain the affected area. It works the body from top down, stimulating circulation and rerouting fluid to healthy pathways, while giving you a gentle workout. Lymphedema is a chronic condition and requires day-to-day self-care. You should do this routine until your swelling is under control, and then move on to address other specific problems, such as pain and flexibility. Return to it whenever you have increased swelling.

You must always remember to wear your sleeve or wrapping while exercising. Never overexert yourself in any way, and do not overtire your arm. At-risk survivors must always be careful (see Eighteen Steps to Prevent Lymphedema on p. 6).

THE LIVING WITH LYMPHEDEMA ROUTINE

◆ The Basic Warm-up (pp. 15–23)
◆ Hawaiian Hula
◆ Close-the-Door Lunges
◆ Overhead Push
◆ Side Arm Swings
◆ Single-Arm Reach
◆ Feel the Water
◆ Finger Rolls
◆ Dance Routine
◆ Healing Visualization

LIVING WITH LYMPHEDEMA 1

HAWAIIAN HULA

Begin here, after doing the Basic Warm-up. The Hawaiian Hula is a graceful dance that gently works your hips and arms as you travel from side to side.

STARTING POSITION: Stand with your feet together and your arms by your sides.

COUNTS: Sixteen.

STEP 1: You're going to move right first. Step out with your right foot, then step your left foot to join it. Let your hips sway. Step to the right again, and this time only touch the ball of your left foot next to it. As you move, brush the air to the right with the backs of your hands as if they were flowing through water.

STEP 2: Now step-together-step-touch to the left, using the same hands.
   Repeat the series.

POINTERS:

◆ Exaggerate the movement of your hips and let your inhibitions go.

◆ Keeping your knees bent allows your hips to move freely.

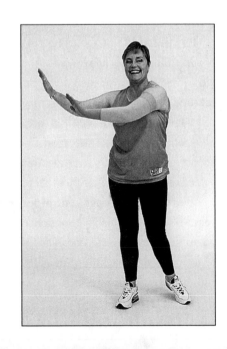

CLOSE-THE-DOOR LUNGES

"I wear my sleeve and glove during the exercises and I seem to be getting better and stronger. The music also makes the routine seem easier. Plus, whenever I need to stop, I just do."
—MONICA, FORTY-THREE

In Close-the-Door Lunges you are working the muscles under your arm. The tendons and scar tissue get a stretch from the wrist to the armpit. Pulsing your hand from a fist to a flexed position and back helps open up the lymphatic system.

STARTING POSITION: Stand with your feet together. Make a fist with your right hand and bend your arm to bring your fist up by your shoulder, as if you're going to box with someone.

COUNTS: Every lunge takes four counts.

STEP 1: Keeping your left leg stationary, lunge your right leg forward about three feet, bending your right knee. As you lunge, your right arm shoots forward and your right hand opens to a flexed position, as if you're slamming a door shut.

STEP 2: Then push off your right heel and bring your leg back to the starting position. At the same time, retract your arm and clench your hand into a fist again.

Do four lunges on the right.

Switch arms and repeat the same series four times on the left.

POINTERS:

◆ Imagine that the door you are slamming is moving farther away from you. This increases the stretch across your upper shoulders and back.

◆ Flex your wrists as much as possible in the lunge position.

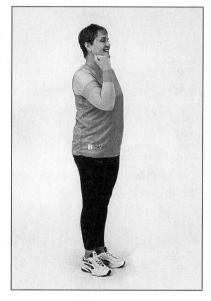

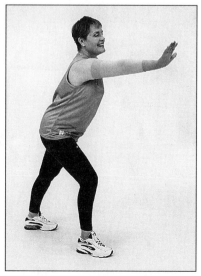

OVERHEAD PUSH

The Overhead Push stretches the scar tissue under your arms where you have had node dissection as well as the muscles along the outside of your arms and the tops of your shoulders. Always work one arm at a time.

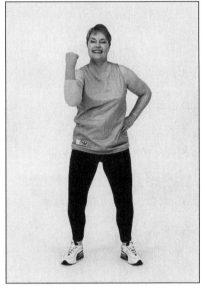

STARTING POSITION: Stand with your feet hip-width apart. Rest your left hand comfortably on your hip. Bend your right elbow so that you bring your right hand up to your right shoulder. Flex your right wrist forward so that your fingers point toward the wall behind you.

COUNTS: Every movement takes four counts.

STEP 1: Bend your knees. As you straighten them, push your right hand up toward the ceiling as if you're a waitress lifting a heavy tray. Keep your arm as close to your head as possible.

STEP 2: Then bend your knees and bring your arm down again. Do not pause at the top.

Repeat four times, then switch arms and do four Overhead Pushes on the left.

POINTER:

◆ Imagine the sensation of carrying a heavy tray. Feel the resistance work your muscles harder and improve the stretch.

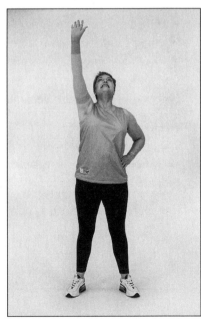

SIDE ARM SWINGS

*"At times my arm feels very heavy, but when I do
the program it feels as light as a feather."*
—NANCY, FORTY-SEVEN

This movement is so much fun that it can help you let go and move a little farther than you might otherwise. It will help stretch out your scar tissue and stimulate your lymphatic fluids.

STARTING POSITION: Stand with your feet hip-width apart and your arms hanging at your sides.

COUNTS: Every swing takes two counts.

STEP 1: Swing both arms easily and freely to the right. Don't strain. As you swing them, shift your weight onto your right foot and allow your left heel to lift off the floor. Follow your hands with your head.

STEP 2: Now swing your arms back down and then up to the left, shifting your weight to your left foot and allowing your right heel to lift off the floor. Follow your hands with your head.

Do eight sets.

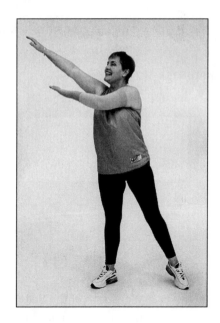

SINGLE-ARM REACH

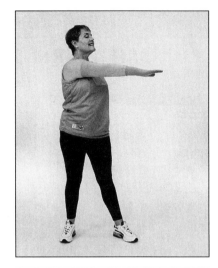

The feeling of the Single Arm Reach is as though someone is pulling your arm and saying, "Come with me!" and you are responding, "No, I don't want to go!" and pulling back. Resistance is what makes the stretch happen. You'll feel it in your shoulder blades and across your rib cage.

STARTING POSITION: Stand with your feet hip-width apart. Your left hand is on your hip.

STEP 1: Reach your right arm to the left as though someone were pulling your arm. Keep your arm straight and pull back with your left shoulder. Then release the tension.

Do four stretches with your right arm.

STEP 2: Now reverse your arms. Repeat the stretch four times with your left arm.

POINTERS:

◆ Keep your elbows straight.

◆ Keep your hips facing front.

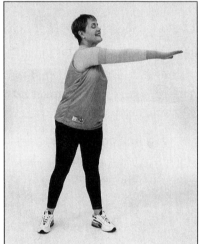

FEEL THE WATER

The arm motions of Feel the Water should be as flowing and easy as though you were underwater.

STARTING POSITION: Stand with your feet hip-width apart.

COUNTS: Every movement takes four counts.

STEP 1: Gently extend your arms forward, keeping them about chest height, while you bend and then straighten your knees.

STEP 2: Now slowly drop your arms down to your sides and then raise them behind you, as high as possible, while you bend and then straighten your knees.

Do four sets.

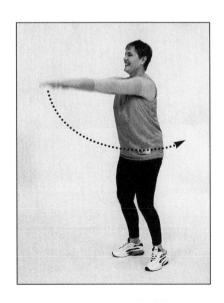

FINGER ROLLS

This movement improves the circulation in your hands, fingers, and arms. It is a terrific antidote for numbness or the feeling of pins and needles. Frequent computer users find it especially helpful.

WHAT YOU NEED FOR THIS EXERCISE: A chair is optional.

STARTING POSITION: Stand or sit. Hold your hands at your shoulders, palms facing forward with your fingers spread wide.

STEP 1: Starting with your little fingers, curl your hands into fists one finger at a time.

STEP 2: Rotate your fists to face you. Then open your hands one finger at a time, again starting with your little fingers.

STEP 3: Then rotate your open palms back to the front.
   Do four sets of Finger Rolls.

POINTER:

◆ Finger Rolls don't have to be done perfectly—unless you're a mime!

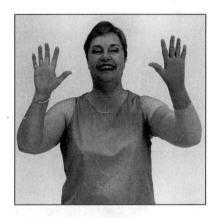

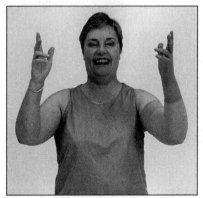

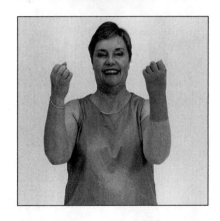

DANCE ROUTINE

"The thought of living with lymphedema used to make me so sad. But dancing in my living room makes me laugh and decreases my pain. Dancing makes me feel so female."

—ROBERTA, FIFTY

This dance routine can help get your lymphatic fluid and your blood circulating. It also makes you smile and feel good. Remember to stop if your arm gets tired; there is always tomorrow.

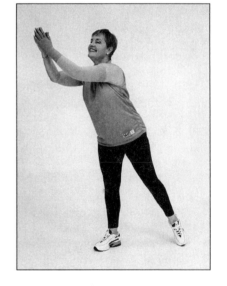

MUSICAL SUGGESTION: Manhattan Transfer, "Java Jive"

STARTING POSITION: Stand with your feet together and your arms hanging by your sides.

LUNGE-POINT: Make a wide step to the right and straighten your knee. Point your left foot and touch it to the left. Hold the position and clap your hands twice to the right. Then transfer your weight to your left leg. Point your right foot and touch it to the right. Hold the position and clap your hands twice to the left.

Do four sets, and then move on to the Showgirl Strut.

THE SHOWGIRL STRUT: Take sixteen steps around the room swinging your arms from right to left overhead like a Las Vegas showgirl with attitude.

Return to the center of the room in preparation for the Charleston.

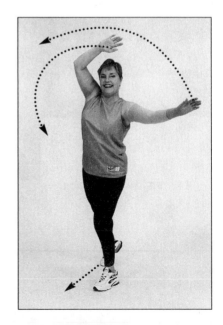

THE CHARLESTON: Step onto your left foot and kick your right leg forward, swinging your arms to the right as you kick. Now step back with your right foot, touch your left foot behind you, and at the same time swing your arms to the left.

Repeat four times. Then come to a stationary position with your feet hip-width apart and your knees slightly bent. Continue with Wash the Windows.

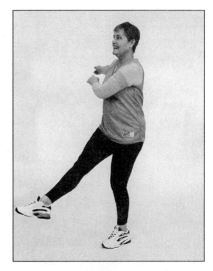

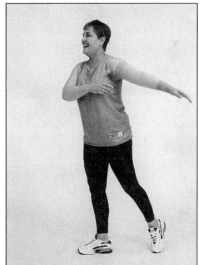

WASH THE WINDOWS: With your wrists flexed, make four big circles in front of your body with your right arm, letting your hips swing freely from side to side. Then make four big circles with your left arm.

Repeat the entire routine from beginning to end until the song ends. Then walk around the room for a few minutes to cool down. Drink some water.

Spend a few quiet minutes doing the Healing Visualization that follows.

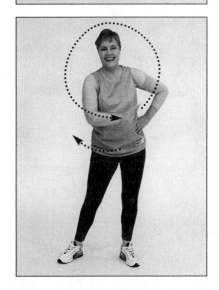

HEALING VISUALIZATION
FOR LYMPHEDEMA

Sit down in a chair and make yourself comfortable. Close your eyes and assess how your body feels right now. Scan your feet, ankles, and legs, then your hands, wrists, and arms. Allow them to relax. Let your belly release. Scan your back, chest, shoulders, neck, and head. Let the hinges of your jaw release. Identify any places of pain and swelling in your body. Tune in to the beating of your heart.

Take long, deep breaths in through your nose and out through your mouth. On every in-breath, visualize a pure blue light filling your body. This light feels cool and it soothes and contracts your swelling as it enters the flow of blood coursing through your veins and arteries.

Imagine yourself swimming easily and freely in the midst of a river. You are as one with the river. Its waters are gentle at first and then become increasingly rapid and turbulent, until they explode over a vast waterfall. You land safely at the bottom and stand jubilantly beneath the falls with your arms outstretched, letting the water wash over you and cleanse your body.

Say three times, "My body circulates fluid freely and easily."

When you feel ready, open your eyes, and come back to the room.

DEVELOPING BALANCE

"I was devastated by the surgery. I just wanted to shrink inside myself.
Focus on Healing was a way to regain my physical balance
so I could get back my emotional balance."

—Judi, fifty-two

Nature made the female body symmetrical. Losing a breast changes the distribution of weight and can affect your sense of balance and control. Prosthetic breasts—breast forms—are designed to match the missing weight, thereby balancing the two sides of the body. However, this is not a perfect science. So whether you choose to wear a breast form or not, you will need to retrain your muscles to accommodate the difference in your body, or you may suffer from neck, shoulder, and back tension. General clumsiness and falling from imbalance can be hazardous, especially to older or inactive women. Exercise is without doubt the best way to restore balance and locate your center of gravity.

For women who have little body awareness, exercise can also instill a new sense of grace.

Delia was a large-busted woman. She wore a 40 DD bra before her mastectomy, and the loss of that single breast threw her horribly off balance. She was left with pain between her shoulder blades, backaches, and poor posture. Her breast form weighed three pounds and felt so uncomfortable that she would always pull it off as soon as she got home. She found herself leaning to one side to compensate and knew she was walking crooked. Tingling and numbness in her hands and feet made it hard to be completely aware of how she was moving. She developed lymphedema in her surgical arm. During chemotherapy she also put on weight, which didn't help the situation. No matter how she tried to adjust on her own, she never felt centered.

Delia then attended a Focus on Healing class for a year. Doing the exercises increased her energy, lessened her symptoms of lymphedema, and improved her range of motion. Most especially the program enabled her to rebalance her body and correct her shoulder placement and posture. Over time her shoulder and back pain went away. Ultimately, for preventive purposes, she opted for elective surgery to remove her other breast. She had two young children and did not want to risk another cancer. One day she may have reconstruction, but for now she frequently practices her exercises and swears that knowledge is power. Understanding and strengthening her body through proper exercise has given her poise and confidence and a new relationship with her body.

BALANCE SPECIFICS FOR SURVIVORS In addition to gently stretching your chest and shoulders, the exercises in this routine are designed to strengthen your lower body, which is your foundation. They also involve shifting your weight from side to side to train you to locate your center of gravity. Some of these exercises are done seated and in some you will use a chair for support. For the others, until you feel confident, please keep a chair nearby in case you're wobbly.

Always wear your breast form while you are exercising. Part of your physical reeducation is learning to accommodate the weight of the prosthetic breast. As you move through the routine, concentrate on keeping your shoulders even and lightly pressed back. In other words, no slouching or tilting. Also, keep your head level and spine straight. Imagine that you are lifting up from your waist.

THE DEVELOPING BALANCE ROUTINE
- The Basic Warm-up (pp. 15–23)
- Mountain High Stretch
- Close-the-Door Lunges
- Single Leg Lifts
- Leg Circles
- Marching in Place
- Calf and Leg Builder
- Hip Tilts
- Side Arm Swings
- Feel the Water
- Step-Touch to the Side
- Step-Touch Forward and Back
- Reach for the Stars
- Chest and Shoulder Stretch
- Dance Routine
- Healing Visualization

MOUNTAIN HIGH STRETCH

Begin here, after doing the Basic Warm-up. Use the Mountain High Stretch to locate your center of balance. Focus on pressing your shoulders down and keeping them level. Your neck and back are forced to compensate when your shoulders are uneven, and that affects your spine, which is what puts you off balance.

STARTING POSITION: Stand with your feet hip-width apart, your arms hanging by your sides.

STEP 1: Bring both arms forward and up, until they are overhead. Hook your fingers together and turn the palms of your hands up to the ceiling. Pull your shoulders up toward your ears. Inhale as you stretch up.

STEP 2: Keeping your fingers interlaced, press your shoulders down hard. Exhale.

Repeat steps 1 and 2 four times.

STEP 3: Next, still keeping your fingers interlaced, tilt your body to the right. Hold and breathe deeply.

STEP 4: Come upright again and tilt to the left. Hold and breathe deeply.

STEP 5: Come upright again and unhook your fingers. With your wrists flexed, slowly lower your arms out to the sides and return them to the starting position.

Do two complete sets.

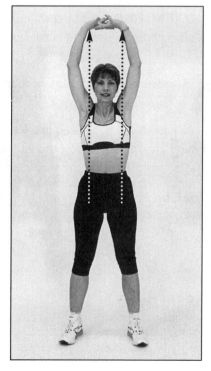

POINTER:

◆ Keep your elbows as straight as possible when your fingers are interlocked.

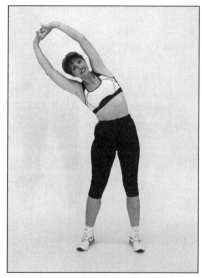

CLOSE-THE-DOOR LUNGES

Close-the-Door Lunges work both the lower and the upper body. After you lunge forward, you have to center your body in order to push back. Therefore it is a wonderful exercise to address balance.

STARTING POSITION: Stand with your feet together. Make a fist with your right hand and bend your arm so that your fist is by your shoulder, as if you're going to box with someone.

COUNTS: Every lunge takes four counts.

STEP 1: Keeping your left leg stationary, lunge your right leg forward about three feet, bending your right knee. As you lunge, your right arm shoots forward and your right hand opens to a flexed position, as if you're slamming a door shut.

STEP 2: Then push off your right heel and bring your leg back to the starting position. At the same time, retract your arm and clench your hand into a fist again.

Do four lunges on the right.

Switch arms and repeat the same series four times on the left.

POINTERS:

◆ Imagine that the door you are slamming is moving farther away from you so that you have to reach your arm out farther. This increases the stretch across your upper shoulders and back.

◆ Flex the wrist of your extended arm as much as possible in the lunge position.

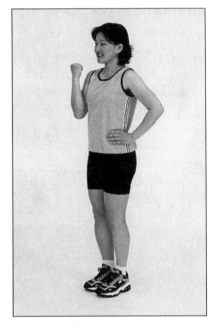

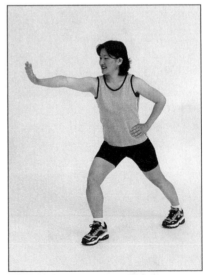

SINGLE LEG LIFTS

*"I didn't even realize my balance was off until
I started the program, and then I was glad to have
a chair next to me to grab on to."*
—TONYA, THIRTY-EIGHT

Single Leg Lifts help you to align your shoulders and center your body.

WHAT YOU NEED FOR THIS EXERCISE: A chair.

STARTING POSITION: Stand with your feet together. Place the chair to your left and hold on to it with your left hand. Your spine is straight and your shoulders are lightly pressed down. Think about pulling your tummy in while you keep breathing.

COUNTS: Every movement takes two counts.

STEP 1: Slowly raise your right leg in front of you and point your toes. Hold for four counts. Then lower it to the starting position and relax your foot. Do four Single Leg Lifts.

STEP 2: Then move to the left of the chair. Do four Single Leg Lifts with your left leg.

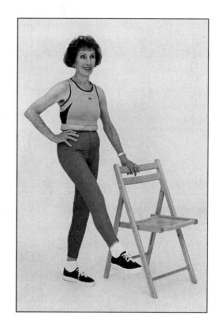

POINTERS:

◆ Concentrating on your quadriceps, the muscles located on the front of your thighs, can help you reap the benefits of this exercise, which works several muscle groups.

◆ Move slowly through the repetitions. It is a simple exercise, but it does a lot.

LEG CIRCLES

In ballet this exercise is called *ronde de jambs,* which is a fancy way of saying leg circles. To do it successfully you have to constantly shift your body and relocate your center of gravity.

WHAT YOU NEED FOR THIS EXERCISE: A chair.

STARTING POSITION: Stand with your feet together. Place the chair to your left and hold on to it with your left hand. You can place your hand on your hips for further stability.

COUNTS: Each Leg Circle takes four counts.

STEP 1: Extend your right leg in front of you and point your right foot so that your toes are touching the floor.

STEP 2: Then draw a slow circle on the floor by taking your foot to the right, then around to the back, and bringing the feet together again in the starting position. Repeat four times.

STEP 3: Now move the chair to your right and hold on to it with your right hand. Make four slow circles on the floor with your left foot.

POINTERS:

◆ Keep your body lifted—holding your stomach in can help.

◆ Check that your shoulders are even.

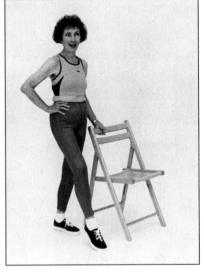

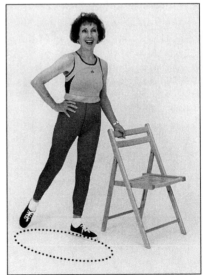

MARCHING IN PLACE

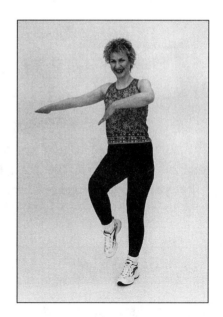

Marching in Place helps you learn to shift your weight equally from side to side, readjusting as necessary to remain stable.

STARTING POSITION: Stand with your feet together and your arms by your sides.

COUNTS: March for sixteen counts.

STEP 1: March your legs, first right and then left, eight times. Swing your arms from side to side as you march to get your blood pumping.

CALF AND LEG BUILDER

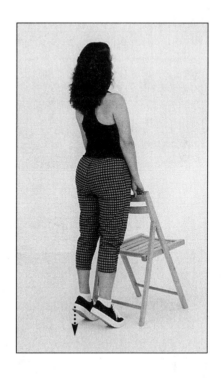

Strong legs equal a strong foundation and, thus, better balance.

WHAT YOU NEED FOR THIS EXERCISE: A supporting chair.

STARTING POSITION: Place the chair in front of you and hold on to it with both hands. Stand at arm's length from the chair with your feet together.

COUNTS: Every movement takes one count.

STEP 1: Rise up onto your toes. Come back down. Do eight times.

POINTERS:

◆ Pull in your stomach and tuck your hips slightly forward.

◆ Remember to press your shoulders down.

HIP TILTS

When you tilt your hips forward you have to relocate your center of gravity. This exercise works your thighs, buttocks, and abdomen . . . and it feels sexy.

STARTING POSITION: Stand with your feet hip-width apart. Your knees are deeply bent. Place your hands on your hips to help you isolate them.

COUNTS: Every Hip Tilt takes four counts.

STEP 1: First do a slow pelvic thrust forward, as you contract your stomach muscles. Then return to center.

STEP 2: Now stick your buttocks out behind you. Return to center.

Do four sets.

POINTERS:

◆ Your chest and shoulders should remain stationary, all the movement is happening in the lower body.

◆ Enjoy yourself!

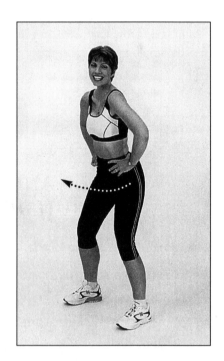

SIDE ARM SWINGS

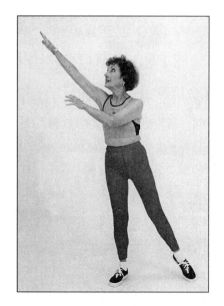

Side Arm Swings can help you learn to accommodate all kinds of shifting movements. Indulge yourself with these slow and easy swings. Allow all your inhibitions to drop away.

STARTING POSITION: Stand with your feet hip-width apart and your arms hanging at your sides.

COUNTS: Every swing takes two counts.

STEP 1: Swing both arms to the right. As you swing your arms, shift your weight onto your right foot and allow your left heel to lift off the floor. Follow your hands with your head.

STEP 2: Now swing your arms back down and then up to the left, shifting your weight to your left foot and allowing your right heel to lift off the floor. Follow your hands with your head.

Do eight sets.

FEEL THE WATER

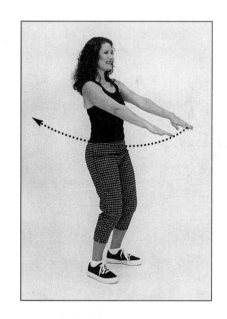

Are you centered enough to move your arms around without losing your balance? Here is a chance to find out. These arm motions should be as flowing and easy as if you were underwater.

STARTING POSITION: Stand with your feet hip-width apart, your arms hanging by your sides.

COUNTS: Each movement takes four counts.

STEP 1: Gently extend your arms forward, keeping them about chest height, while you are first bending and then straightening your knees.

STEP 2: Now slowly drop your arms down to your sides and then raise them behind you, as high as possible, while you are first bending and then straightening your knees.

Repeat twice.

STEP-TOUCH TO THE SIDE

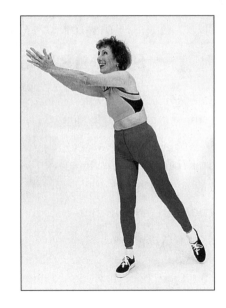

Here's a chance to shift your weight from side to side while having fun and dancing. You go girl!

STARTING POSITION: Stand with your feet together. Your arms are by your sides.

COUNTS: Every movement takes one count.

STEP 1: Step to the right.

STEP 2: Touch your left foot to the side while swinging your arms to the right and clapping your hands at shoulder height. Turn your head toward your hands as you clap.

STEP 3: Now step to the left.

STEP 4: Touch your right foot to the side while swinging your arms to the left and clapping your hands at shoulder height. Turn your head toward your hands as you clap.
   Do four sets.

STEP-TOUCH FORWARD AND BACK

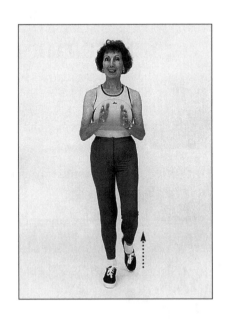

You are still dancing with this exercise. If you feel wobbly doing these steps, you may opt to march in place instead.

STARTING POSITION: Stand with your feet together, your arms at your sides.

COUNTS: Every movement takes one count.

STEP 1: Step forward with the right foot.

STEP 2: Then bring your left foot forward and touch your right foot while clapping your hands.

STEP 3: Now step back onto your left foot.

STEP 4: Bring your right foot back to touch your left foot while clapping your hands.
   Do four sets.

POINTER:

◆ Be careful during this exercise since you're shifting your weight more than in most.

REACH FOR THE STARS

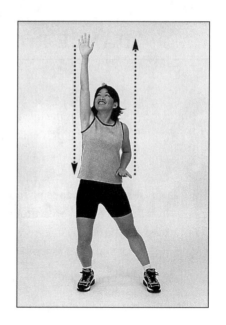

Have you been favoring one side of your body more than the other since your treatment? Stretching both sides equally can help restore your equilibrium.

STARTING POSITION: Stand with your feet hip-width apart. Your hands are on your hips.

COUNTS: Every reach takes four counts.

STEP 1: Reach your right arm up, as though you are trying to touch a star. Then reach farther for a second count. Lower your right hand to your hip on two counts.

STEP 2: Now reach up the same way with your left arm.
Do four sets.

CHEST AND SHOULDER STRETCH

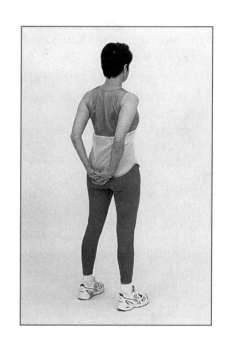

The Chest and Shoulder Stretch builds strength and flexibility in your shoulders, chest, and arms, and therefore promotes proper body centering.

STARTING POSITION: Stand with your feet hip-width apart. Interlace your fingers behind your lower back with your palms facing up.

STEP 1: Straighten your arms as much as you can and inhale deeply while lifting your chest up and forward. Press your shoulders all the way back and down. Exaggerate the position by thinking about your shoulder blades coming together. Hold the position for two more deep breaths in and out.

STEP 2: Keeping your hands clasped, relax the position and slump your shoulders forward. Exhale.
Repeat the stretch four times.

DANCE ROUTINE

"This dance routine opens me up. Afterward I stand taller and feel better. It gets my blood going."
—JENNIFER, SEVENTY-FIVE

This is a variation of a tap dancing routine. All the women in my classes love it. They put on an attitude and get into the act. Feel free to keep a chair nearby in case you want to dance around it and lean on it for stability. Remember, you are sensational!

MUSICAL SUGGESTION: "One" from the musical *A Chorus Line.*

STARTING POSITION: Stand with your legs together. Your hands are on your hips.

SHUFFLE STEP: Bend your right knee, placing it against your left knee as if you were a flamingo. Then straighten your knee and bring your right foot forward, brushing the ball of your right foot against the floor as you go. Then brush it back, bending your right knee back into its former position. Then stamp your right foot on the floor.

Switch legs and repeat these movements with your left leg.

Do four sets, ending with your feet together in preparation for the Traveling Tap Step.

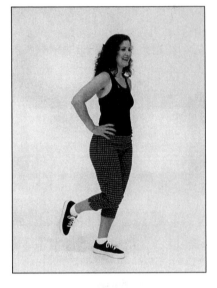

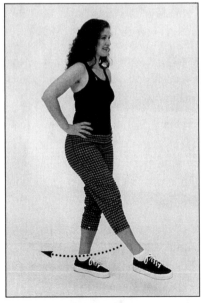

TRAVELING TAP STEP: Smack the ball of your right foot a little in front of you, as if there's a tap on the bottom of your shoe. Then put your right heel down. Do the same tap step on the left so that you began to travel forward. Swing your arms from side to side as you step.

Do four sets, and then continue with Toe Taps.

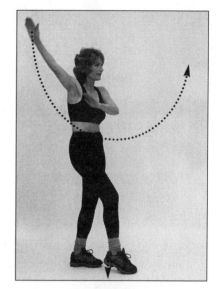

TOE TAP: Tap your right foot to the front. Tap it to the right side. Tap it behind you. Then bring your feet together.

Repeat with your left foot.

Do two sets.

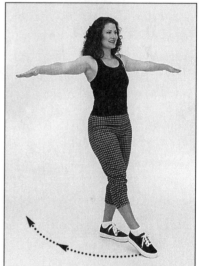

STEP-KICK: Step to the right with your right foot. Then kick to the right with your left leg so that it crosses over your right. Now immediately step to the left with your left foot, and then kick to the left with your right leg. Clap your hands every time you kick your legs.

Do four sets.

When you've finished, walk around the room for a minute, or walk in place, to cool down. Take a drink of water. Then spend a few minutes doing the Healing Visualization that follows.

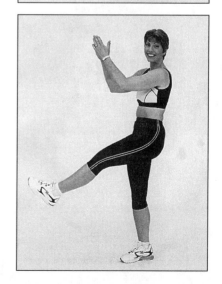

HEALING VISUALIZATION
FOR BALANCE

Take a seat and make yourself comfortable. Close your eyes. Let gravity pull down on you and relax your muscles. Scan your feet, ankles, and legs, then your hands, wrists, and arms. Allow them to relax. Let your belly release. Scan your back, chest, shoulders, neck, and head. Allow them to relax. Identify whether the right and left sides of your body feel the same or different. Accept what you find without changing anything.

Breathe in a deep, rich indigo blue light that fills you from the core with peace. On every exhalation this blue light grows larger, into a cloud of serenity that envelops you and everything around you.

Imagine that you can see within this blue cloud an orange-gold tightrope stretching out in front of you. You are holding a long, narrow pole in your hands. You step confidently and lightly across the entire length of the high wire in perfect balance, arriving safely on the other side.

Say three times, "I am graceful and nimble and poised."

Take as many trips across the wire as you like and then, when you feel ready, open your eyes and return to the room.

MENOPAUSE

"Your doctor may not mention menopause to you, because he is treating your cancer and focused on keeping you alive. That may be all you care about for a while, too. But menopause often goes with the territory and it is up to you to ask questions. Ask, ask, ask."

—*Mary, forty-one*

Menopause is a phase of life that all women experience eventually. You may even have been going through menopause naturally at the time of your cancer diagnosis. In any case, menopause can also be induced by certain medications or the shock of chemotherapy and radiation on a woman's system. One younger woman in my class thought she was having a nervous breakdown when she started having regular crying jags. She asked her gynecologist and he confirmed that she was in early menopause. As a result of cancer treatment, there have even been cases of women who have already passed through the change of life who suddenly experience their menopausal symptoms for a second time.

Since postcancer drugs like tamoxifen affect your hormones, they can trigger menopause or increase symptoms you're already experiencing, such as hot flashes and mood swings. Other side effects of menopause can include weight gain and a loss of sex drive, muscle tone, and flexibility. Exercise is an antidote to all of these side effects. Movement helps you release stress-related hormones, which would otherwise be stored in your body's tissues, and gives you an endorphin rush that makes you feel much better. It is also a way to moderate unwanted weight gain.

Mary was only twenty-eight when she had a lumpectomy and follow-up chemotherapy and radiation. Nine years later her doctor removed a tumor in her left lung and she went on tamoxifen. At age forty another tumor was removed from her right lung and her doctor began giving her regular shots of Lupron, a drug that turns off the ovaries, because estrogen has been known to speed the growth of cancer cells. In addition, she was required to take a daily dose of Megace to control her hormone levels. As a result, her appetite soared and she gained an unhealthy amount of weight; so, after five months, her doctor took her off the Megace pills. A few months later she found herself in the midst of menopause and also stopped taking Lupron. One of her doctors had mentioned in passing that she might experience early menopause, but when it happened she was still taken off guard.

Mary felt extremely moody and suffered from hot flashes. The hot flashes were bad, yet she found the emotional side effects even more diffi-cult to bear. The worst thing about her menopause was her lack of sexual desire. At first she was hesitant to say anything about it. Then she was glad she did because she found a physician who prescribed a medication that helped restore her libido without using hormones. During her difficult transition Focus on Healing relieved her stress, helped her handle her emotions, and helped her stabilize her weight. More important, the program helped her regain a sense of control over her life and put some joy back in her days. She loves Focus on Healing so much that she became a certified instructor and now teaches classes in New Jersey.

Whether induced menopausal symptoms are permanent may depend on where you currently are in your life cycle. Younger women usually begin menstruating again later, though not always. While menopause may not have been part of your current plans, it is manageable and inevitable and you will get through it, I promise. Women have been thriving past menopause for centuries.

MENOPAUSE SPECIFICS FOR SURVIVORS It is important, during and after menopause, to make exercise a regular part of your life. Keeping limber and strengthening your muscles have been proven to help prevent osteoporosis, the loss of bone density that is common in postmenopausal women. Regular exercise also helps you maintain your ideal weight and increases your energy. This routine is designed to alleviate the mood swings and depression that may accompany menopause. Its sensual hip movements can also help you feel sexual and vibrant.

THE MENOPAUSE ROUTINE

◆ The Basic Warm-up (pp. 15–23)
◆ Mountain High Stretch

- ◆ Small Arm Circles
- ◆ Hip Tilts
- ◆ Hip Swings
- ◆ Gentle Body Twists
- ◆ The Showgirl Strut
- ◆ Wash the Windows
- ◆ Lower Body Ultimates (pp. 169–174)
- ◆ Building Strength (pp. 177–182)
- ◆ Dance Routine
- ◆ Healing Visualization

MOUNTAIN HIGH STRETCH

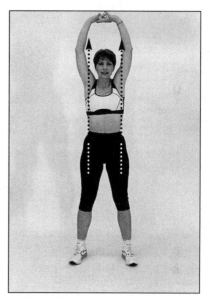

Begin here, after doing the Basic Warm-up. It is very important to elongate your scar tissue, especially since those emotional mood swings can result in slouching and poor posture.

STARTING POSITION: Stand with your feet hip-width apart, your arms hanging by your sides.

STEP 1: Bring both arms forward and up, until they are overhead. Hook your fingers together and turn the palms of your hands up to the ceiling. Pull your shoulders up toward your ears. Inhale as you stretch up.

STEP 2: Keeping your fingers interlaced, press your shoulders down hard. Exhale.

Repeat steps 1 and 2 four times.

STEP 3: Next, still keeping your fingers interlaced, tilt your body to the right. Hold and breathe deeply.

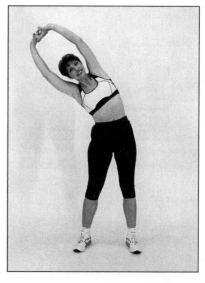

STEP 4: Come upright again and tilt to the left. Hold and breathe deeply.

STEP 5: Come upright again and unhook your fingers. With your wrists flexed, slowly lower your arms out to the sides and return them to the starting position.

Do two complete sets.

POINTER:
- ◆ Keep your elbows as straight as possible when your fingers are interlocked.

115

SMALL ARM CIRCLES

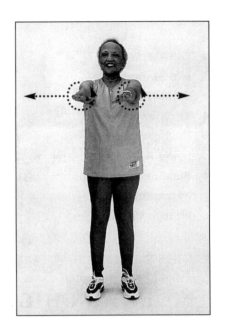

You can start rebuilding your muscular strength with these isometric arm circles that tone your shoulders and upper arms.

STARTING POSITION: Stand with your feet hip-width apart. Your arms are extended straight out in front of you at shoulder height. The palms of your hands are facing the floor.

COUNTS: Each Small Arm Circle takes one count.

STEP 1: Circle your arms outward in small, tight circles eight times. Then circle them inward in tight circles eight times.

STEP 2: Next, open your arms out to the sides. Make eight tight circles backward, and then eight forward.

HIP TILTS

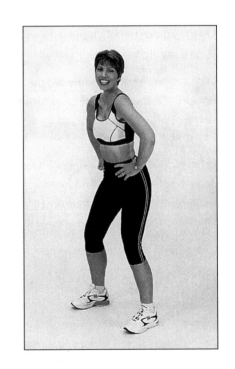

Hip Tilts allow you to feel sexy . . . and at the same time you find your center of gravity.

STARTING POSITION: Stand with your feet hip-width apart. Your knees are deeply bent. Place your hands on your hips to help you isolate them.

COUNTS: Every Hip Tilt takes four counts.

STEP 1: First do a slow pelvic thrust forward, as you contract your stomach muscles.

Return to center.

STEP 2: Now stick your buttocks out behind you. Return to center.

Do four sets.

POINTER:

◆ Your chest and shoulders should remain stationary—all the movement is happening in your lower body.

HIP SWINGS

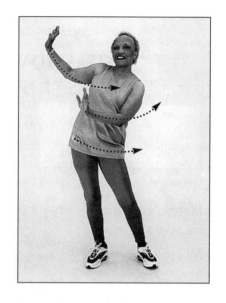

"After chemotherapy and radiation I started experiencing mood swings and didn't know why. I would cry, then be fine, be sad, and then be fine. Then I started on tamoxifen and got hot flashes along with the mood swings, and I thought I was going crazy. It turns out I was going through my menopause symptoms all over again. My doctor gave me Lorazepam for the anxiety and Megestrol for the hot flashes, and I increased my exercise time to every other day. As soon as I understood why I was feeling the way I was—and that I was not crazy— I started feeling better. Now I feel wonderful."
—BETTY, SIXTY-THREE

STARTING POSITION: Stand with your feet hip-width apart and your knees slightly bent.

COUNTS: Every movement takes two counts.

STEP 1: Swing your hips slowly from right to left and back again eight times. Allow your arms to swing freely from side to side.

GENTLE BODY TWISTS

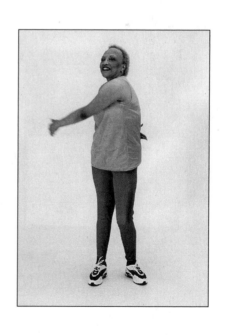

Gentle Body Twists wake up the spine and stretch the muscles below your shoulder blades. It is important to move slowly and stay relaxed while doing them since it can feel intense. You may choose to skip this exercise if you have a bad back.

STARTING POSITION: Stand with your feet hip-width apart. Your arms are raised out to the sides at shoulder height.

COUNTS: Every twist takes four counts.

STEP 1: Turn your upper body to the right so that you get a nice twist and stretch along your spine. Let your arms be relaxed and flop comfortably around you.

STEP 2: Gently rotate back to center and then turn to the left. Do four sets.

THE SHOWGIRL STRUT

I always get a little wild during this exercise—after all, who's watching? Swinging your arms helps accelerate the release of endorphins. More important, however, this exercise is truly feminine, which is such a gift during the time of menopause.

STARTING POSITION: Stand with your feet together and raise your arms overhead.

COUNTS: Every movement is one count.

STEP 1: Step to the right, swinging your arms from left to right overhead like a Las Vegas showgirl with attitude.

STEP 2: Then touch your left foot to the side.

STEP 3: Now step to the left, swinging your arms overhead from right to left.

STEP 4: Then touch your right foot to the side.
   Do eight sets.

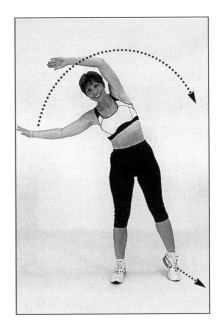

WASH THE WINDOWS

Let everything out emotionally and physically with this exercise. It improves your range of motion, gets your endorphins going, and helps relieve stress. One survivor in my class told me, "I have not smiled and had so much fun or felt feminine in a long time. If I washed windows like this at home my husband would love it. Maybe I will."

STARTING POSITION: Stand with your feet hip-width apart and your knees slightly bent.

COUNTS: Every circle takes four counts.

STEP 1: Keeping your wrist flexed, make four large circles in front of your body with your right arm, as though you were washing a giant window. Let your hips swing freely from side to side.

STEP 2: Now make four large circles with your left arm.

At this point in the Menopause program, you should add on the "Lower Body Ultimates" (beginning on page 169) and "Building Strength" exercises (beginning on page 177). Afterward, continue with the Dance Routine on the next page.

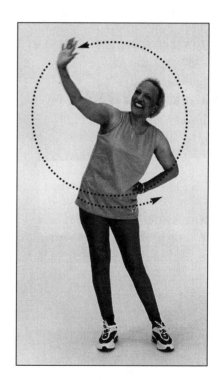

DANCE ROUTINE

When I was going through menopause my husband would enter our house slowly, since he never knew exactly who would greet him. I guess I had a few different personalities in those days. Thankfully, my mood swings have settled down. I have to tell you though, I have been a dancer all my life, and dance class was my salvation. I could express my emotions openly there and release all the pent-up stress I was carrying around. On the dance floor I didn't have to apologize for drama or passion and I felt sensual, earthy, and connected to my body, like a powerful woman.

So, with this dance routine, build up a sweat and really go for it. The routine relieves stress, cools hot flashes, helps you feel feminine, and should give you a happy boost. Have fun!

MUSICAL SUGGESTION: The Bee Gees, "Hand Jivin'"

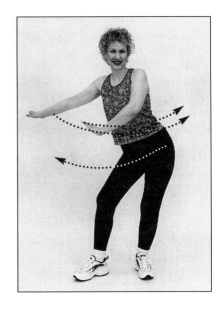

CHUBBY CHECKER TWIST: Bend your knees and twist your lower body first to the right and then to the left while swinging your arms naturally in the opposite direction.

Do eight sets, and then move on to the Showgirl Strut.

THE SHOWGIRL STRUT: Step to the right, swinging your arms from left to right overhead like a Las Vegas showgirl with attitude. Then touch your left foot to the side. Step to the left, swinging your arms overhead from right to left. Then touch your right foot to the side.

Do eight sets. Then come back to a stationary position and lower your arms in preparation for the Hawaiian Hula.

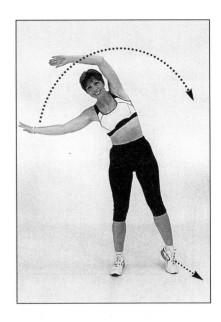

THE HAWAIIAN HULA: Step out to the right with your right foot, and then bring your left foot over to join it. Let your hips sway in an exaggerated motion. Step to the right again, and then touch the ball of your left foot next to your right foot. As you take your steps, brush the air to the right with the backs of your hands as if they were flowing through water.

Now travel left, step-together-step-touching with the same hand gesture.

Do four sets. Then come to a stationary position with your feet hip-width apart and your arms down by your sides in preparation for Arm Flops.

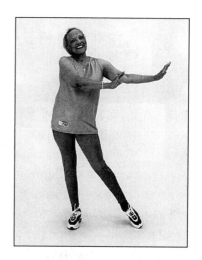

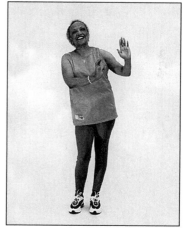

ARM FLOPS: Reach your arms up, and then flop them down behind your head. Reach them up again, and flop them down to your sides. Swing your hips from right to left while doing your arm movements.

Do four Arm Flops.

Keep doing the whole routine from beginning to end until the song ends. Then take a walk around the room for a few minutes and drink some water.

Spend a few minutes doing the Healing Visualization that follows.

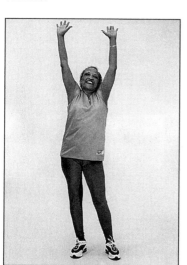

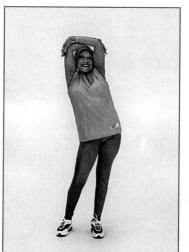

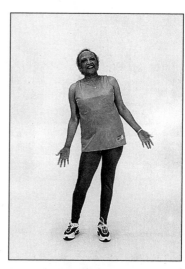

HEALING VISUALIZATION
FOR MENOPAUSE

Take a seat and make yourself comfortable. Close your eyes and begin scanning your body. Direct your attention to your feet, ankles, and legs, then your hands, wrists, and arms. Let your belly be released. Feel your head floating on the top of your spine. Move your attention to your back, chest, and shoulders, then your neck and scalp. Let your jaw and the muscles of your face hang loose. Tune in to your emotions. Trust that whatever feelings are coming up are acceptable. They are only messages from your nervous system. Allow them simply to be there.

Breathe deeply and rhythmically and relax. Imagine that you are being filled with a pure silvery-blue healing light.

Now imagine that it is a clear and starry night out, and you are floating on your back in a lake of serenity. It's a balmy summer evening and a gentle breeze kisses your face. You are weightless and completely supported. As you gaze into the sky a meteor shower begins, and you let your irritability fly away on a shooting star. It passes brightly through the heavens, and then is gone. On another star you send away your hot flashes.

Keep releasing your symptoms one at a time—seeing them fly through the night sky like shooting stars—until none are left. Only you are there in the stillness of nature.

Say three times, "I am relaxed, calm, and cool."

When you are done, open your eyes and return.

EXPLORING YOUR FEMININITY

"First you lose your breast, and then you lose your hair.
You lose a lot—just being a woman."

—Kathy, fifty-five

Sexuality is not just about physical appearance, it's also about how we feel inside. The image of being wounded by cancer is reinforced by the missing breast, the weight gain, and the hair lost to chemotherapy. What makes each of us feel feminine is highly individual, and often determined by our culture and circumstances. And how we grieve our losses depends on the meaning we attach to different parts of our bodies. Losing eyelashes or pubic and underarm hair can be just as devastating to some women as losing the hair on top of their head. They all can impact our sense of femininity, our libido, and our sexual confidence.

It is important to remind ourselves that no matter our outward appearance, we are whole women. Sexuality comes from how we feel inside ourselves, our vibrancy. You may look and seem healthy and fine to the outside world, to your friends, family, and mate, while below the surface you have lost your desire and your sense of sensuality. Exercise, especially dance steps and gestures, can help reawaken your connection to your femininity.

Kathy had been married for only four months when she was diagnosed with cancer at age fifty-two. Many women in her immediate family were survivors before her and she had seen the challenges firsthand. She could imagine what the diagnosis would mean for her and her husband. The same day they chopped down their first Christmas tree, Kathy underwent a bilateral mastectomy. Afterward she went through a course of chemotherapy. Her husband was wonderful; he helped her get through the bad days that followed. Nonetheless it was hard for her when she stood undressed in front of him or the mirror. In losing her breasts and her hair, she felt stripped of her femininity.

Kathy had always especially loved her thick hair. It made her feel beautiful and womanly. Now it was gone and no one could tell her if it would grow back strong and healthy. She wrestled internally with the decision to have reconstructive surgery, until a close friend who had it done four years earlier lifted her shirt to show Kathy the positive results that could be achieved. Her friend joked, "See, now you can look like Barbie, too!"

Kathy had reconstruction and physical therapy until her insurance coverage ran out. Then she joined a Focus on Healing class to keep working on her range of motion. There she reconnected with the little girl inside her who had always felt pretty and special in her dance class. She learned to swing her hips without feeling embarrassed in a way that she had forgotten she could do. Whenever the music starts she lets herself drift and be carried away into a fantasy as she dances. Kathy always wears lovely lacey underwear that makes her feel feminine and ladylike. When her hair came back in, she grew it as long as she could and has vowed to keep it that length forever.

FEMININITY SPECIFICS FOR SURVIVORS This dance routine is designed to help you feel sexy and free and rebuild confidence in your body. Use this as an opportunity to explore your sensuality by letting your hips sway and emphasizing the feminine gestures. In dancing you can be whoever you want to be. No one is watching or judging you. As long as you warm up properly and take care not to do rapid pushing or pulling movements, you are perfectly safe.

EXPLORING YOUR FEMININITY ROUTINE:
◆ The Basic Warm-up (pp. 15–23)
◆ Mountain High Stretch
◆ Overhead Side Stretch
◆ Hip Swings
◆ Step-Touch with Hand Shakes
◆ Hawaiian Hula
◆ Reach for the Stars
◆ Close-the-Door Lunges
◆ Side Lunges
◆ Big Hug
◆ The Leg Routine
◆ Dance Routine
◆ Healing Visualization

MOUNTAIN HIGH STRETCH

Begin here, after doing the Basic Warm-up. Posture is significant both to your emotional makeup and your physical well-being. Stretching and lengthening your torso in this exercise feels good and will help you stand taller and straighter.

STARTING POSITION: Stand with your feet hip-width apart, your arms hanging by your sides.

STEP 1: Bring both arms forward and up, until they are overhead. Hook your fingers together and turn the palms of your hands up to the ceiling. Pull your shoulders up toward your ears. Inhale as you stretch up.

STEP 2: Keeping your fingers interlaced, press your shoulders down hard. Exhale.

   Repeat steps 1 and 2 four times.

STEP 3: Next, still keeping your fingers interlaced, tilt your body to the right. Hold and breathe deeply.

STEP 4: Come upright again and tilt to the left. Hold and breathe deeply.

STEP 5: Come upright again and unhook your fingers. With your wrists flexed, slowly lower your arms out to the sides and return them to the starting position.

   Do two complete sets.

POINTER:

◆ Keep your elbows as straight as possible when your fingers are interlocked.

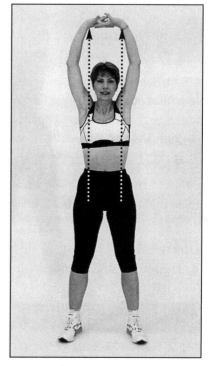

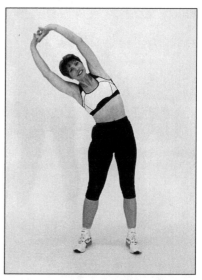

OVERHEAD SIDE STRETCH

I find it hard to feel graceful and feminine when my muscles are tight. Stretching out your muscles and scar tissue by gently elongating your sides, torso, and underarms releases that sense of constriction.

STARTING POSITION: Stand with your feet hip-width apart, your arms hanging at your sides with the palms facing inward.

STEP 1: Swing your right arm slowly out to the side and up over your head. Your palm should be facing out. Gently tilt your body to the left and reach to the left with your right arm. Hold this position for two deep breaths in and out.

STEP 2: Return your body to an upright position and bring your right arm back down, making a slow, reaching arc.

Repeat the stretch on your left side.

Do two more stretches on each side.

POINTERS:

◆ Keep your palms facing outward even at the height of the stretch.

◆ Be gentle and move slowly.

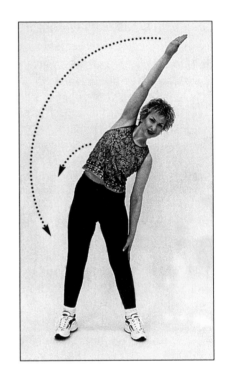

HIP SWINGS

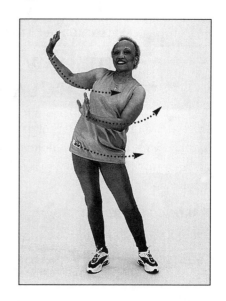

What could be sexier than to let your hips and arms swing with the music? When was the last time you "rocked"?

STARTING POSITION: Stand with your feet hip-width apart and your knees slightly bent.

COUNTS: Every swing takes two counts.

STEP 1: Swing your hips slowly from right to left and back again eight times. Allow your arms to move naturally from side to side; there's no specific arm motion you must follow.

POINTER:

◆ Relax and enjoy yourself. There are no hidden cameras taking candid pictures.

STEP-TOUCH WITH HAND SHAKES

"When I hear the music and move to it, I feel so sexy. I just let it all go and move. It is wonderful to feel in control of my life again."
—WENDY, FIFTY-NINE

This exercise not only gives you a total body workout, it allows you to move your hips and body like the sexy and feminine woman you are!

STARTING POSITION: Stand with your feet together, your arms by your sides.

COUNTS: Every movement takes one count.

STEP 1: Step to the right. Then bring your left foot over and touch it to the side. Shake your hands constantly while you step-touch, as though they are wet and you don't have a towel.

STEP 2: Now step to the left. Then touch your right foot to the side. Do four sets.

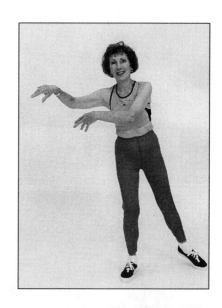

THE HAWAIIAN HULA

The Hawaiian Hula is a graceful dance that gently works your hips and arms as you travel from side to side. Imagine that a warm tropical breeze is blowing across your body as you dance in the moonlight.

STARTING POSITION: Stand with your feet together and your arms by your sides.

COUNTS: Every movement takes one count.

STEP 1: First you're going to move to the right. Step to the side with your right foot, then bring your left foot across to join it. Let your hips sway. Step to the right again, and touch the ball of your left foot next to your right foot. As you move, brush the air to the right with the backs of your hands as if they were flowing through water.

STEP 2: Then step-together, step-touch to the left, using the same hands.

Do eight complete sets.

POINTER:

◆ Exaggerate the movement of your hips and let your inhibitions go. Keeping your knees bent allows your hips to move freely.

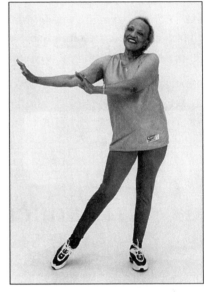

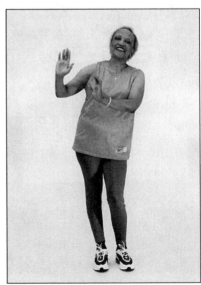

REACH FOR THE STARS

Reach for the stars. Reach for your dreams. I know you've got some!

STARTING POSITION: Stand with your feet hip-width apart. Your hands are on your hips.

COUNTS: Every reach takes four counts.

STEP 1: Reach your right arm up, as though you are trying to touch a star. Then reach farther for a second count. Lower your right hand to your hip on two counts.

STEP 2: Now reach up the same way with your left arm.
   Do four sets.

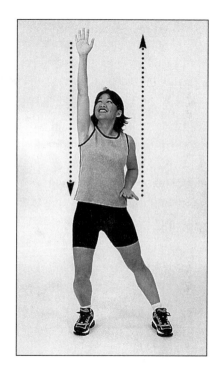

CLOSE-THE-DOOR LUNGES

When was the last time you could be dramatic in closing a door? This is your big opportunity to be a diva. Exaggerate the move.

STARTING POSITION: Stand with your feet together. Make a fist with your right hand and bend your arm so that your fist is by your shoulder, as if you're going to box with someone.

COUNTS: Every lunge takes four counts.

STEP 1: Keeping your left leg stationary, lunge your right leg forward about three feet, bending your right knee. As you lunge, your right arm shoots forward and your right hand opens to a flexed position, as if you're slamming a door shut.

STEP 2: Then push off your right heel and bring your leg back to the starting position. At the same time, retract your arm and clench your hand into a fist again.

Do four lunges on the right.

Switch arms and repeat the same series four times on the left.

POINTERS:

◆ Imagine that the door you are slamming is moving farther away from you so that you reach your arm out farther. This increases the stretch across your upper shoulders and back.

◆ Flex the wrist of your extended arm as much as possible in the lunge position.

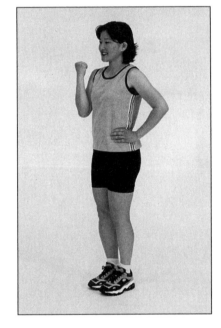

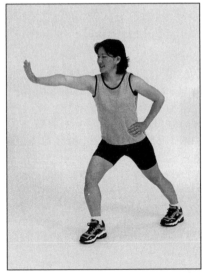

SIDE LUNGES

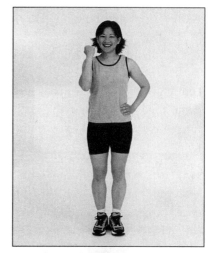

Side Lunges are similar to Close-the-Door Lunges. Be dramatic. Have fun.

STARTING POSITION: Stand with your feet together. Make a fist with your right hand and bend your arm so that your fist is by your right shoulder, as if you're going to box with someone. Place your left hand on your hip.

COUNTS: Every Side Lunge takes four counts.

STEP 1: Keeping your left leg stationary, lunge your right leg to the side about two feet, bending your right knee. As you lunge, your right arm shoots to the side and your right hand opens to a flexed position. Look at your hand.

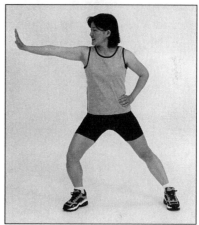

STEP 2: Now push off your right heel and bring your leg back to the starting position. At the same time, retract your arm and clench your hand into a fist again.

Do four lunges on the right side.

Switch arms and repeat the same series four times on the left.

BIG HUG

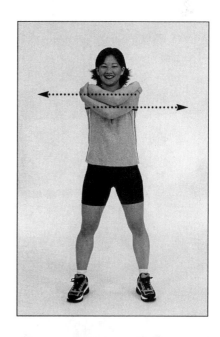

One of our primary needs as human beings is the need for touch. When was the last time you were hugged? Give yourself a Big Hug now, and then go find someone else and share some affection.

STARTING POSITION: Extend your arms out to your sides at shoulder height.

STEP 1: Wrap your arms around yourself in a Big Hug with your right arm on top.

STEP 2: Extend your arms to the sides again. Then hug yourself with your left arm on top.

THE LEG ROUTINE

I put together this leg workout specifically to help you feel feminine. Toned calves and thighs are especially attractive features—and you can achieve them through these exercises. So go for it.

STARTING POSITION: Stand with your feet together. At first, keep your hands on your waist throughout the routine. Later, once you are confident about the leg movements, you may let your hands move freely in any way that is comfortable.

FORWARD STEP-TOUCH: First you're going to travel forward. Step forward with your right foot, then your left foot, and then your right foot again. Then touch your left foot next to the right.

Do four sets, and then do the Backward Step-Touch.

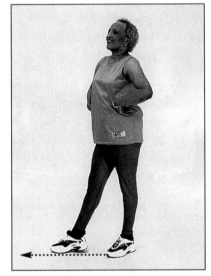

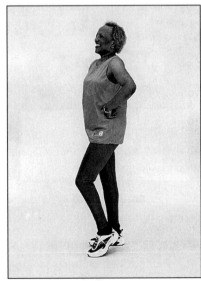

BACKWARD STEP-TOUCH: Now you're going to travel backward. Step back with your right foot, then your left foot, and then your right foot again. Then touch your left foot next to your right.

Do four sets, and then continue with Step-Kicks.

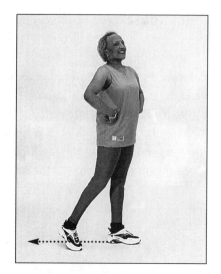

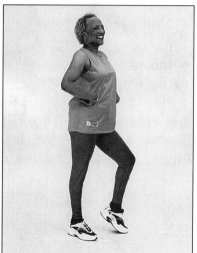

STEP-KICKS: Next you're going to travel sideways. Step onto your right foot and kick to the right with your left leg as you clap your hands. Now step onto your left foot and kick to the left with your right leg as you clap your hands.

Do four sets, and then come to a stationary position. Separate your feet by a distance of two to three feet. Your toes are pointed outward. Place your hands on your hips. Continue with the Thigh Toner.

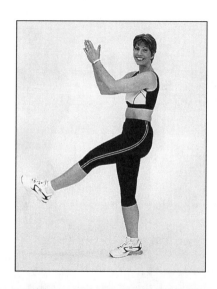

THIGH TONER: Bend and straighten your knees, going down on one count and coming up on one count.

Repeat three times.

Now begin a fourth Thigh Toner, but this time, go down and hold the position for eight counts. Then straighten.

Your ultimate goal is to do four complete sets. Begin with one or two sets.

After you come up the last time, extend your arms to the sides and immediately begin the Tango Slide.

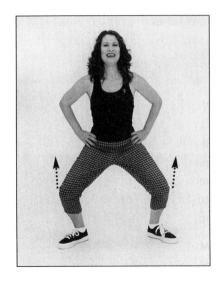

TANGO SLIDE: Lunge your right leg about a foot to the right and bend your right knee. Next, slide your left foot along the floor until it touches your right foot and then straighten your right leg. Now slide your left foot up your right calf to your right knee. Then lunge your left foot out to the left side and bend your left knee. Do the Tango Slide with your right foot.

Do two sets.

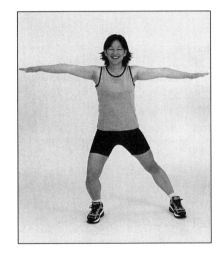

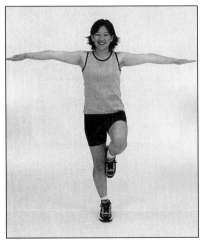

DANCE ROUTINE

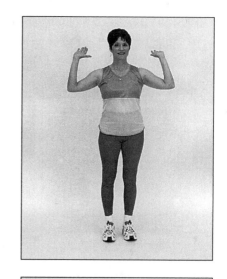

When I came home from the hospital I didn't feel the same and I didn't want my husband to look at me because I was different. It took awhile to restore my confidence. Dancing holds a special place in my heart because it helped me get past my fears, reclaim my body, and rekindle my spirit. Once I discovered that I could still feel pleasure dancing, it was much easier to accept myself as I now was.

MUSICAL SUGGESTION: "The Girl from Ipanema" from the CD *Mambo Mambo*.

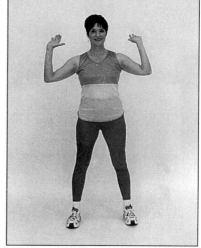

STEP-TOGETHER-STEP-TOUCH: You're going to travel right. Start with your feet together. Bend your elbows and raise your hands to your shoulders. Step out and shift your weight onto your right foot. Now bring your left foot beside it. Step out again onto your right foot. This time, touch your left foot beside the right without placing your weight on it. As you touch your left foot down, push your hands straight up over your head.

Bring your hands back to shoulder height as you begin to travel left, stepping out with your left foot. Do the same series in reverse: step-together-step-touch. Push your hands to the ceiling as you touch your right foot.

Continue right away with the Showgirl Strut.

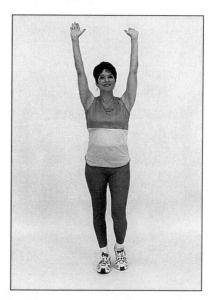

THE SHOWGIRL STRUT: Step to the right, swinging your arms from left to right overhead like a Las Vegas showgirl with attitude. Then touch your left foot to the side. Step to the left, swinging your arms overhead from right to left. Then touch your right foot to the side.

Do eight sets.

Then come to a stationary position with your feet hip-width apart and your arms down by your sides in preparation for Arm Flops.

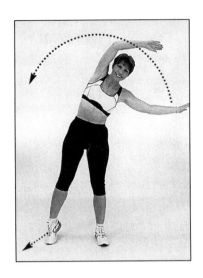

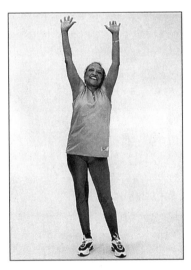
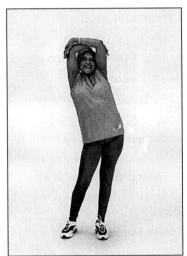
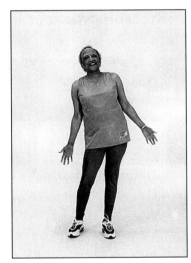

ARM FLOPS: Swinging your hips from right to left, reach your arms up, and then flop them down behind your head. Reach them up again, and flop them down to your sides.

Repeat four times. Then bring your feet together and your hands up to your shoulders in preparation for the Mambo.

THE MAMBO: Step forward onto your right foot. Then pick up your left foot and put it back down. Bring your right foot back to the left. Hold for a beat.

Now step backward onto your left foot. Step in place with your right foot. Bring your left foot forward to rejoin your right foot. Hold for a beat.

Do four sets of Mambos.

Continue doing the whole routine from beginning to end until the song is over. Then take a short walk around the room to cool down. Have a drink of water.

Enjoy the following Healing Visualization. It's one of my favorites!

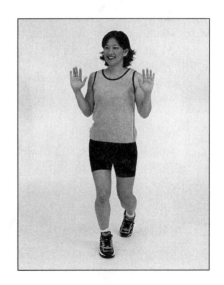

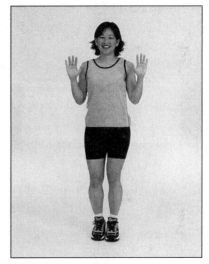

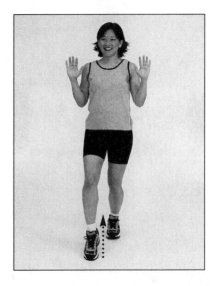

HEALING VISUALIZATION
FOR FEMININITY

Sit down in a chair and make yourself comfortable. Close your eyes and begin to breathe deeply. Tune in to the sensations of your physical body. How does your lower body feel? Are the muscles in your feet, ankles, and legs relaxed? Relax your calves and thighs. Scan through your abdomen. Feel your breath moving into your belly and expanding into your lower back. Relax your hips. Imagine that you are a tree rooted into the center of the earth. Feel how you are connected to the earth, how you are a part of nature.

Next scan your fingers, hands, wrists, and arms. Let the muscles in your upper body release. Feel your chest rise and fall with the breath and your back open. Your neck is long and proud; your shoulders are relaxed. Release any tension in your jaw, forehead, and around your eyes.

As you breathe in, breathe in a passionate, fiery red color. It fills you with intense vitality. As you breathe out, breathe out sparks and glowing embers.

Imagine that you are wearing fabulous clothes, and look so stunning and sexy that every eye follows you as you enter a ballroom. You are magnetic. A handsome dance partner awaits you across the floor. You slowly move toward him as the band strikes up a tango. You embrace and dance, lunging and entwining, never letting your eyes separate. Every move you make is mirrored. You understand each other perfectly. Your pulse is pounding. The music speaks the language of your soul. There has never been another night like this one. You are energized and aware of your deepest animal instincts.

Say three times, "I am a beautiful, sexy, feminine goddess."

When you are ready, open your eyes.

AFTER RECONSTRUCTION

"Stay positive. Think on the bright side and surround yourself with positive people. Take every day as a gift from God. Smell the flowers, breathe in the air, enjoy the raindrops, and keep smiling."

—*Betty, sixty-three*

*Y*ou deserve to feel good about yourself and your body. Some survivors elect to have breast reconstruction following their mastectomies. The decision to have reconstructive surgery is a deeply personal one. You may have it at the same time as your original surgery or months or years afterward. There are several different procedures, including implants and back or abdominal flaps; the kind that is right for you is something you need to discuss with your surgeon.

When Betty was done with her reconstructive surgery she finally felt complete. From the time she was initially diagnosed with cancer the year before, her three daughters and husband had given her unconditional love and support, which made the treatment much easier to bear. The first day she went for chemo her husband even stepped out and got his head shaved as a gesture of solidarity. It gave her a good laugh and also touched her heart. There was never any pity, only genuine understanding. However, since her mastectomy she had truly missed her breast. Now, after reconstruction, she felt emotionally restored.

Betty was confident about her decision. To make a better match, she had a breast reduction done on her remaining breast, and then a *latissimus dorsi* flap reconstruction on the site of her missing breast. A tattoo of a nipple was added as a finishing element. Her doctors were excellent and carefully explained every step in the process. As a result, her reconstruction was an uplifting experience.

For a few weeks Betty had to be careful to keep the surgical sites dry and clean, and to not lie on her side. She was not very sore; there was only mild pain. She was advised not to exercise until the skin was healed and the swelling went down. Her arm and chest became a little stiff from the inactivity. But she was soon able to begin Focus on Healing classes, through which she was able to increase her range of motion. Three years later, she finds that doing the program three times a week prevents the same stiffness and soreness from returning. To this workout schedule she has added several hours each week spent walking briskly on a treadmill.

Structured exercise is enormously important when coping with the aftermath of reconstruc-

tion, just as it is following initial breast surgery. Areas of your body that are healing from tissue and muscle grafting, or expansion from saline implantation may be extremely sensitive and tight. You may develop more scar tissue. Gentle stretching can reduce your pain and help you restore and maintain your flexibility both in the short-term and for the rest of your life.

POSTRECONSTRUCTION SPECIFICS FOR SURVIVORS This routine is designed for the survivor who has recently undergone a breast reconstruction. Some surgeons recommend that their patients wait a full year after reconstruction to begin stretching. Others believe it is okay to exercise after just one month. Because every surgery and every healing process is unique, I advise you to seek your doctor's opinion and advice prior to starting this program.

Depending upon your individual circumstances and your doctor's approval, you should use this routine for approximately two months, until you are ready to move on to the other routines in this book, such as "Restoring Flexibility" (p. 29) and eventually the Upper Body Ultimates in Part Three, "The Ultimate Movements" (p. 156–158).

Many women who have been through reconstructive surgery struggle with issues of balance. The weight of a new breast may differ from your original breast and your muscles need to learn to compensate for the change. If you have this problem, after working through "Restoring Flexibility," please be sure to spend some time on "Developing Balance" (p. 100).

Another issue that often accompanies reconstruction is numbness. As you are healing, you may find that you have lost some or all of the sensation in your chest. Therefore it is critical that you move with caution. Be sure to warm up properly with the Basic Warm-up and go gently through this routine, until some or all of your sensation returns.

Especially if you have had an abdominal flap procedure, hold your stomach in as you work through the exercises in this chapter. You should aim to build strength slowly.

THE AFTER RECONSTRUCTION ROUTINE
◆ The Basic Warm-up (pp. 15–23)
◆ Wall Push-ups
◆ Wall Stretch
◆ Shoulder Blade Squeeze
◆ Arm Rotations
◆ Overhead Side Stretch
◆ Circle the Moon
◆ Bicep Curls
◆ Climbing the Ladder
◆ Dance Routine
◆ Healing Visualization

WALL PUSH-UPS

Begin here, after doing the Basic Warm-up. With this exercise you have a choice. You can either do Wall Push-ups in the corner of a room, which is optimum, or facing a flat wall.

STARTING POSITION: Stand two feet away from the wall with your legs hip-width apart. Place your arms at chest height on the wall and your hands about a foot apart. If this is an uncomfortable distance, move closer. For a greater chest stretch, move your hands farther apart. Turn your fingers slightly toward each other. If this position hurts your wrists, find a compensating position that suits your special needs. Turn your hands as upright as necessary to eliminate any wrist discomfort.

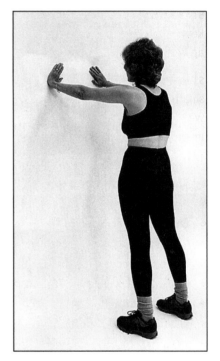

COUNTS: Every Wall Push-up takes four counts.

STEP 1: On a slow count of two, bend your arms and lean into the wall, bringing your face about four inches away from it. Be careful not to sway your back or cave in. Your body should be as straight as a wooden board.

STEP 2: Push back on another count of two to return to the starting position.

Begin with two push-ups. Then gradually increase the number you're doing from two to twelve over the course of a month or two. Whenever you feel strong enough to do more repetitions, add two push-ups. You should stay at the same level for at least three more workouts before adding on again.

POINTERS:

◆ Be careful not to sway your back or cave in. Your body should be as straight as a wooden board.

◆ Stop if you feel pain in your arms. You can relieve some of the strain on your arms by lifting your elbows and turning your fingertips to face each other.

◆ Concentrate on tightening your buttocks.

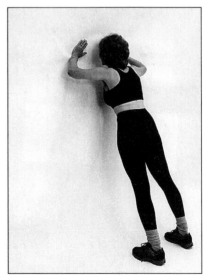

WALL STRETCH

This is a simple, gentle stretch for your shoulders, chest, and upper back. You can control the intensity of the movement by moving your hands up or down the wall.

STARTING POSITION: Stand a few inches away from the wall. Reach both arms over your head and place your hands flat against the wall.

STEP 1: Keeping your hands where they are, bend your knees slightly and gently try to walk your fingers a little farther up the wall. Keep your knees bent, hold the stretch for two deep breaths in and out, and then straighten your legs. Repeat.

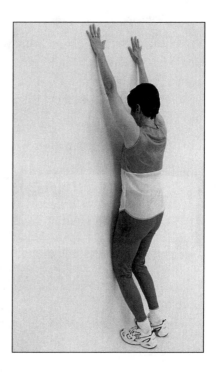

SHOULDER BLADE SQUEEZE

After reconstructive surgery your chest may feel numb. Shoulder Blade Squeezes can help open this area without unknowingly pulling or tearing tissue. When I was young, girls would do this exercise and chant, "I must, I must, I must increase my bust." Now, years later, we can use it to help stretch scar tissue around our new busts.

STARTING POSITION: Stand with your feet hip-width apart. Bend your elbows and lift them to shoulder height so that your hands are in front of your chest, fingertips touching. Your palms are facing the floor. Your shoulders are dropped comfortably and even.

COUNTS: Each movement takes two counts.

STEP 1: Squeeze your shoulder blades together. Allow your fingertips to separate and your elbows to rotate behind you.

STEP 2: Return to the starting position. Repeat three times.

STEP 3: Now open your arms straight out to the sides keeping them at shoulder height and squeezing your shoulder blades together. Return to the starting position. Only do this movement once.

Repeat the entire series three times.

POINTERS:

◆ Keep your shoulders pressed lightly down.

◆ As you pull your elbows back, imagine your chest expanding gently forward.

◆ Stop whenever your arms feel fatigued. Do not overexert.

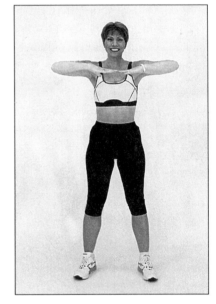

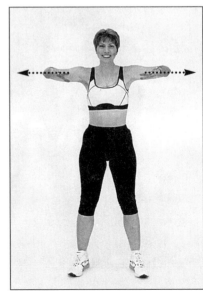

ARM ROTATIONS

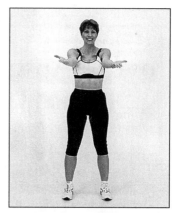

One of my students loves her new breast. She told me she feels like she's thirty again, especially since they fixed her other fifty-six-year-old breast to be thirty, too! This exercise keeps your shoulders loose and prevents the tightening of scar tissue. I should mention that some women find this a tough exercise, so please be careful and stop if you feel any discomfort. Remember, you are the best monitor of your own abilities.

STARTING POSITION: Stand with your feet hip-width apart. Your arms are extended out in front of you at chest height, palms facing the ceiling. Your elbows remain straight throughout this program.

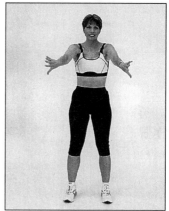

COUNTS: Every movement takes two counts.

STEP 1: Turn your palms inward to face each other.

STEP 2: Then turn them downward.

STEP 3: Turn them outward so that the backs of your hands face each other.

STEP 4: Then turn them downward again.

STEP 5: Turn them inward.

STEP 6: Then turn them upward again to the starting position. Repeat four times.

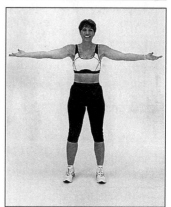

STEP 7: Next, move your arms out to the sides at shoulder height with your palms still facing the ceiling.

STEP 8: Turn them forward.

STEP 9: Then turn them downward.

STEP 10: Turn them backward.

STEP 11: Then turn them up again, allowing your shoulder to roll forward.

STEP 12: Reverse direction and turn them backward again.

STEP 13: Turn them downward.

STEP 14: Turn them frontward.

STEP 15: Then turn them upward again. Repeat four times. Do four sets.

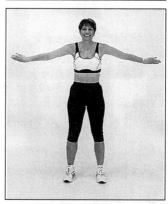

OVERHEAD SIDE STRETCH

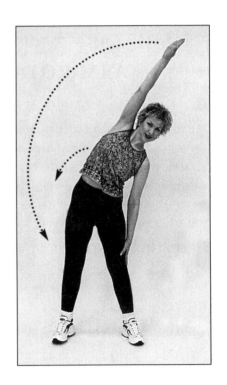

These stretches slowly and gently elongate the muscles along your side, arm, and torso. You need to be gentle with scar tissue after surgery. One survivor told me that after her reconstructive surgery she literally had no feeling from her neck to her waist. She was afraid she would hurt herself going back to her regular activities because she wouldn't know if she tore something. Now, after doing this program, she is ready to go back to her normal exercise routine, but she always does a presport warm-up.

STARTING POSITION: Stand with your feet hip-width apart; your arms hanging by your sides with the palms facing inward.

STEP 1: Swing your right arm slowly out to the side and up over your head. Your palm should be facing out. Gently tilt your body to the left and reach to the left with your right arm. Hold this position for two deep breaths in and out.

STEP 2: Return your body to an upright position. Then bring your right arm back down, making a slow, reaching arc.

Repeat the stretch on your left side.

Do two more stretches on each side.

POINTERS:

◆ Keep your palm facing outward even at the height of your stretch.

◆ Be gentle and move slowly.

CIRCLE THE MOON

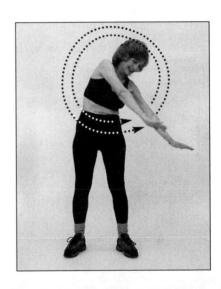

This exercise is designed to help you regain your range of motion, stretch scar tissue, and loosen up any tightness in the area of your chest.

STARTING POSITION: Stand with your feet hip-width apart, and your arms hanging by your sides.

COUNTS: Every circle takes eight counts.

STEP 1: Both arms move together. Imagine that you're holding a small beach ball between your hands. Circle them to the right, then up overhead, and then down to the left. Repeat.

Then circle your arms twice in the opposite direction.

POINTER:

◆ Move very slowly.

BICEP CURLS

"A free tummy tuck," said one of my new students, as she proudly showed me her new breast and stomach after her abdominal flap procedure.

WHAT YOU NEED FOR THIS EXERCISE: An elastic workout band.

STARTING POSITION: Step on one end of your band, either with the heel or the ball of your right foot. Hold the other end of the band in your right hand. The palm of your hand is turned forward, and the end of your band dangles from the little finger side of your fist. Lock your right arm tight against the side of your body. Your wrist should be straight, not flexed during this exercise and you should stand tall.

COUNTS: Four counts to curl and four counts to release.

STEP 1: Bend your right elbow and slowly bring your hand up to your shoulder. Return slowly to the starting position. Repeat four times.

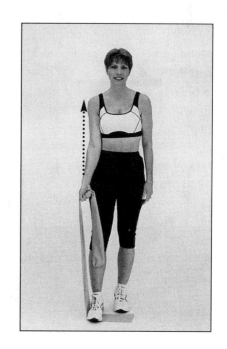

STEP 2: Switch the elastic band to your left hand and foot. When you are ready, repeat the Bicep Curl four times with your left arm.

POINTER:

◆ I find that I have more balance and strength when I put the foot on my working side a little bit behind the other. But this is a matter of preference. You should take the stance that is most comfortable for you.

CLIMBING THE LADDER

As you do this exercise pretend that you have a spongy rubber ball in each hand and that you are alternately squeezing and releasing them. This boosts your circulation.

STARTING POSITION: Stand with your feet hip-width apart. Make loose fists with your hands and place them at your waist.

COUNTS: Every movement takes two counts.

STEP 1: First, reach your right arm forward at waist height. Open your hand, bring your right shoulder forward, and bend your right knee, shifting your weight to your right leg.

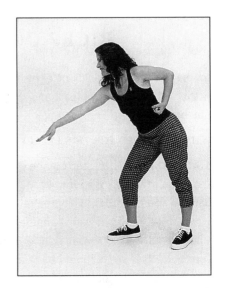

STEP 2: Now reach your left arm forward at waist height, bend your left knee, bring your left shoulder forward, and open your left hand. Your weight shifts to your left leg. At the same time, straighten your right knee and pull your right hand back in to your waist, making a fist again.

STEP 3: Reverse the arms, shoulders, and legs again—reaching your right hand forward to shoulder height, with your left hand coming back to your waist, where you make a fist.

STEP 4: Reverse the movements again. Reach your left arm out to shoulder height and pull your right hand back to your waist and make a fist.

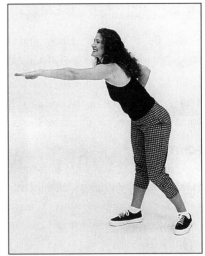

STEP 5: Reverse the movements again. This time, though, reach your right arm forward to face height. Pull your left hand back to your waist.

STEP 6: Then do the reverse with your left arm to face height and your right arm coming into your waist.

STEP 7: For the next four beats, alternate reaching above your head first with the right arm and then with the left arm, bending the same knee as the arm that is reaching upward. Continue opening your hand as your arm reaches full extension and closing your hand as it comes down to your waist.

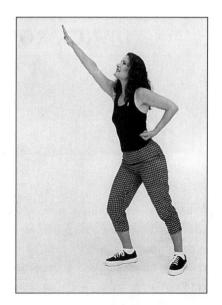

STEP 8: Now repeat the same actions you made going up, this time moving downward. First reach your hands to face height, then reach them to shoulder height, and finally to waist height.
Complete two whole series.

POINTER:
◆ This series of movements must be performed slowly to protect you from injury.

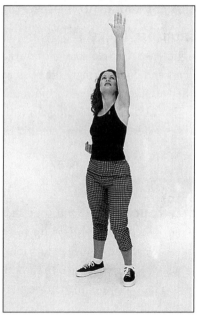

DANCE ROUTINE

*"The best thing is that now that I have had reconstruction,
I don't need to worry about my prosthetic breast
shifting around anymore."*
—DONNA, FORTY-THREE

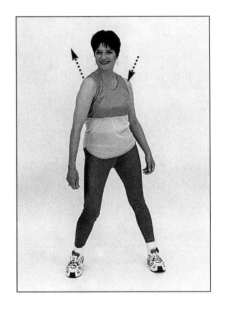

Dancing can help tremendously as you recover from your reconstructive surgery. Switching your weight fluidly from foot to foot especially helps you learn how to balance with the weight of your new breast. It is also an opportunity to feel graceful and celebrate your femininity and your new body.

MUSICAL SUGGESTION: Jennifer Lopez, "Let's Get Loud."

SHOULDER SHAKE: Begin with your feet together. Step to the right. Then, for two counts of music, shake your shoulders forward and back as many times as you can, first right then left. Then step your left foot to join your right foot.

Now travel left, stepping out with your left foot. Do the same series in reverse. Do two sets, and then continue with the Step-Touch.

STEP-TOUCH: Step to the right. Touch your left foot to the side while swinging your arms up to the right and clapping your hands. Now step to the left and touch your right foot to the side while swinging your arms to the left and clapping your hands.

Do four sets, and then move on to the Showgirl Strut.

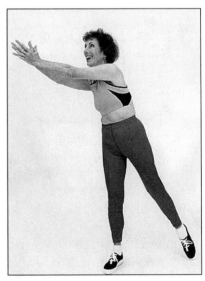

THE SHOWGIRL STRUT: Step to the right, swinging your arms from left to right overhead like a Las Vegas showgirl with attitude. Then touch your left foot to the side. Step to the left, swinging your arms overhead from right to left. Then touch your right foot to the side.

Do eight sets.

Come to a stationary position in preparation for Reach for the Stars. Your legs are hip-width apart and your hands are on your hips.

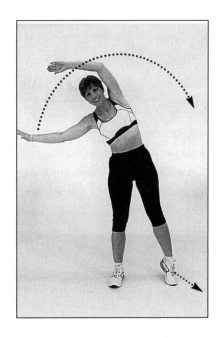

REACH FOR THE STARS: Reach your right arm up, as though you are trying to touch a star. Then reach farther for a second count. Lower your right hand to your hip on two counts.

Now reach up the same way with your left arm.

Repeat four times.

Do the whole routine as many times as you can from start to finish until the song ends. Then walk around the room for about a minute to slow your heart rate. Take a drink of water.

Spend a few quiet minutes doing the Healing Visualization that follows.

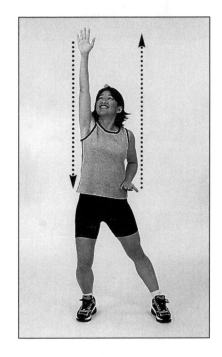

HEALING VISUALIZATION
FOR AFTER RECONSTRUCTION

Take a seat and make yourself comfortable. Close your eyes. Now tune in to your body. Are your feet, ankles, and legs relaxed? How about your hands, wrists, and arms? Do you feel any tightness in your upper body? How about your face? Allow your jaw and the muscles in your back, shoulder, and neck to release. Breathe deeply and slowly in through your nose and out through your mouth. Become aware of your feelings and sensations. Allow your thoughts to still.

Imagine yourself entering a temple. Within the temple is a warm bathtub filled with lovely scented water. Disrobe, step in, and allow yourself to sink back into the soothing water. Candles are lit and golden light is flickering around you. There is beautiful music playing softly in the background. In this sacred place you have no cares and no troubles. You have all the time in the world.

When you are ready, ask your intuition whether there is any particular way or anything you need in order to be kind to yourself right now—anything at all. Receive the answer.

Say three times, "My body is stronger and healthier every day. I accept and nurture myself through the healing process."

In your own time, allow your eyes to open.

PART THREE

The Ultimate Movements

THE ULTIMATE MOVEMENTS

"Doing Focus on Healing opens me up.
It has helped me stand taller and feel better."

—*Beth, fifty-six*

The Ultimate Movements are the thirty-minute-long program at the heart of the Focus on Healing system. Once you are pain-free and have achieved a full range of motion, I recommend that you do this full program three times a week for the rest of your life. Reaching this level of fitness is your long-term goal.

The Ultimate Movements are divided into three main sections, which you will then follow with a five-minute dance routine and healing visualization.

These are:

- ◆ **UPPER BODY ULTIMATES:** fourteen standing exercises targeted to your arms, shoulders, chest, back, and neck. The standing series gently stretches your scar tissue and improves your circulation.
- ◆ **LOWER BODY ULTIMATES:** eight seated exercises targeted to your stomach, buttocks, and leg muscles. The seated series helps you establish a strong physical foundation and improves your balance.
- ◆ **BUILDING STRENGTH:** seven isometric exercises targeting specific muscles in the upper body (incorporates the use of an elastic exercise band).

If you have specific problems that would prevent you from completing the Ultimate Movements at the present time, such as pain, frozen shoulder, or lymphedema, to name a few, please return to Part Two, "Adjusting to the Needs of Your New Body." The routines there are designed to lead you to accomplish the Ultimate Movements.

Some survivors have told me that they prefer to do the program in segments; for example work out with the Upper Body Ultimates in the morning and the Lower Body Ultimates in the afternoon, or on alternating days. That's okay. However, I encourage you to do all three sections at some point during the week. If you are going to separate them, remember that you must prepare yourself each time by doing the Basic Warm-up. You can do the Ultimate Dance Routine and Healing Visualization following any part of the program.

MUSICAL SUGGESTION: Once you've completed the Basic Warm-up, put on some faster-tempo music—anything that inspires you and makes you feel glad to be alive.

Now you're ready to begin the Ultimate Movements.

MOUNTAIN HIGH STRETCH

Begin here, after doing the Basic Warm-up. The Mountain High Stretch gently elongates scar tissue and helps prevent frozen shoulder. It is also a great way to relax your neck and release the tension that so many of us carry in our shoulders. Because your hands can swell after you've had lymph nodes removed, every few hours that you're stationary you should lift your arms and use this stretch to get your circulation moving. You can do it in a car when you're stuck in traffic. You can also do it at your desk in an office.

STARTING POSITION: Stand with your feet hip-width apart, your arms hanging by your sides.

STEP 1: Bring both arms forward and up, until they are overhead. Hook your fingers together and turn the palms of your hands up to the ceiling. Pull your shoulders up toward your ears. Inhale as you stretch up.

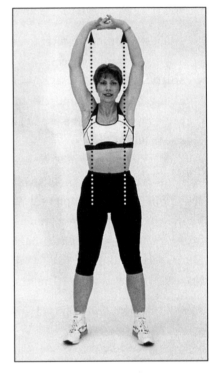

STEP 2: Keeping your fingers interlaced, press your shoulders down hard. Exhale.

Repeat steps 1 and 2 four times.

STEP 3: Next, still keeping your fingers interlaced, tilt your body to the right. Hold and breathe deeply.

STEP 4: Come upright again and tilt to the left. Hold and breathe deeply.

STEP 5: Come upright again and unhook your fingers. With your wrists flexed, slowly lower your arms out to the sides and return them to the starting position.

Do two complete sets.

POINTER:

◆ Keep your elbows as straight as possible when your fingers are interlocked.

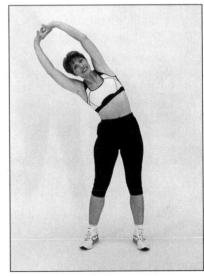

WALL PUSH-UPS

I love Wall Push-ups because I cannot do regular push-ups on the floor anymore as a result of my surgery. These are safer because they put less stress on the area that was treated. But even though it's less demanding than the original, this exercise works exactly the same muscles. The goal is to expand your chest and at the same time strengthen your back and shoulders, arms, stomach, buttocks, and legs. You also get a good hamstring stretch as you lean forward.

You have a choice. You can do Wall Push-ups in the corner of a room, which is optimum, or facing a flat wall.

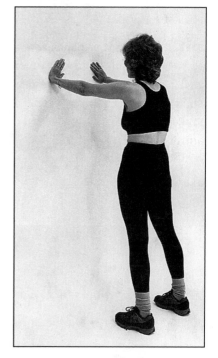

STARTING POSITION: Stand two feet away from the wall with your legs hip-width apart. Place your arms at chest height on the wall and your hands about a foot apart. If this is an uncomfortable distance, move closer. For a greater chest stretch, move your hands farther apart. Turn your fingers slightly toward each other. If this position hurts your wrists, find a compensating position that suits your special needs. Turn your hands as upright as necessary to eliminate any wrist discomfort.

COUNTS: Every Wall Push-up takes four counts.

STEP 1: On a slow count of two, bend your arms and lean into the wall, bringing your face about four inches away from it. Be careful not to sway your back or cave in. Your body should be as straight as a wooden board.

STEP 2: Push back on another count of two to return to the starting position.

Begin with two push-ups. Then gradually increase the number you're doing from two to twelve over the course of a month or two. Whenever you feel strong enough to do more repetitions, add two push-ups. You should stay at the same level for at least three more workouts before adding on again.

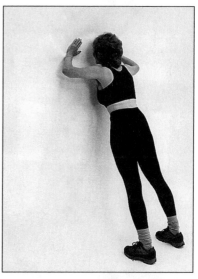

POINTER:

◆ Concentrate on tightening your buttocks.

WALL STRETCH

This is a simple, gentle stretch for your shoulders, chest, and upper back. You can control the intensity of the movement by moving your hands up or down the wall.

STARTING POSITION: Stand a few inches away from the wall. Reach both arms over your head and place your hands flat against the wall.

STEP 1: Keeping your hands where they are, bend your knees slightly and gently try to walk your fingers a little farther up the wall. Hold the stretch for two deep breaths in and out. Then straighten your legs.

Repeat.

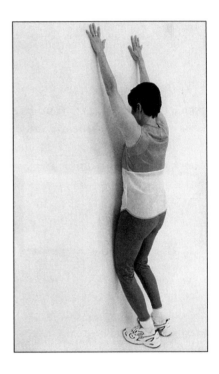

OVERHEAD PUSH

The Overhead Push helps stretch the scar tissue under your arms if you've had node dissection as well as the muscles along the outside of your arms and the tops of your shoulders. Always work one arm at a time.

STARTING POSITION: Stand with your feet hip-width apart. Rest your left hand comfortably on your hip. Bend your right elbow so that you bring your right hand up to your right shoulder. Flex your right wrist backward so that your fingers point toward the wall behind you.

COUNTS: Every movement takes four counts.

STEP 1: Bend your knees. As you straighten them, push your right hand up toward the ceiling as if you're a waitress lifting a heavy tray. Keep your arm as close to your head as possible.

STEP 2: Then bend your knees and bring your arm down again. Do not pause at the top.

Repeat four times, then switch arms and do four on the left.

POINTER:

◆ Imagine the sensation of carrying a heavy tray; feeling the resistance makes your muscles work harder and improves the stretch.

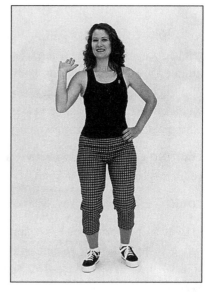

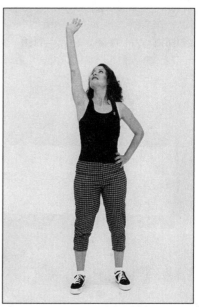

SIDE ARM SWINGS

"Believe in yourself! You will have your life back and you can be stronger and better."
—NANCY, FORTY-SEVEN

You may be frightened of getting hurt and therefore hold yourself back. Doing Side Arm Swings can help you move beyond self-imposed limits, let go of your inhibitions, and gain freedom of movement. So relax and have fun! Give yourself permission to indulge in these slow, easy movements. This exercise should feel pleasurable, rather than stressful or difficult in any way.

STARTING POSITION: Stand with your feet hip-width apart and your arms hanging at your sides.

COUNTS: Every swing takes two counts.

STEP 1: Swing both arms easily and freely to the right. As you swing them, shift your weight onto your right foot and allow your left heel to lift off the floor. Follow your hands with your head.

STEP 2: Now swing your arms back down and up to the left, shifting your weight to your left foot and allowing your right heel to lift off the floor. Follow your hands with your head.

   Do eight sets.

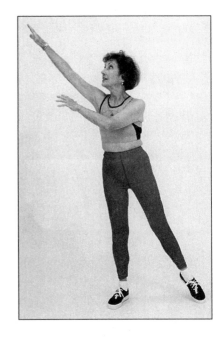

HIP SWINGS

"Live life with a sense of joy.
Don't worry about tomorrow, enjoy today."
—ANGEL, THIRTY-TWO

The point of Hip Swings is to loosen your hips and get them ready to work harder. Like Side Arm Swings, I find that this releases me emotionally as well as physically.

STARTING POSITION: Stand with your feet hip-width apart and your knees slightly bent.

COUNTS: Every swing takes two counts.

STEP 1: Swing your hips slowly from right to left and back again eight times. Allow your arms to swing freely from side to side; there's no specific arm motion you must follow.

POINTER:
◆ Relax and enjoy yourself. There are no hidden cameras taking candid pictures.

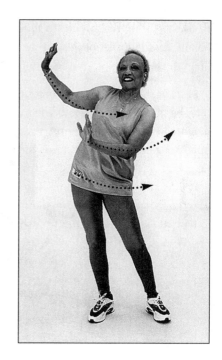

THE CRAWL

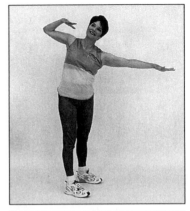

The next three exercises are taken right from the swimming pool. They may remind you of your first swim lessons—before the instructor let you in the water. The good news is that you don't have to put on a bathing suit. Instead, you'll imagine the resistance of the water.

STARTING POSITION: Stand with your feet hip-width apart. Your arms should be straight out in front of your body at shoulder height—or as high as you can lift them.

COUNTS: Every arm circle takes eight counts.

STEP 1: To do the Crawl, your arms must cycle independently. Lower your right arm down to your side, then bend your right elbow and bring the arm up to shoulder height. From shoulder height, continue the movement by extending the arm straight up in the air.

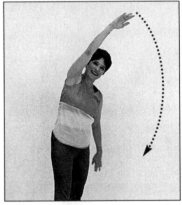

STEP 2: At the same time, bring your left arm down to your side, then bend the left elbow and bring your left arm up to shoulder height. As the left arm is rising, circle the right arm forward and down to the starting position. As the left arm continues straight up into the air, lower your right arm to your side.

Circle both arms four times. Turn your head to the right as your right hand reaches your shoulder and then turn it to the left as your left hand reaches your shoulder. Your movements are continuous and flowing. Try to find a steady rhythm.

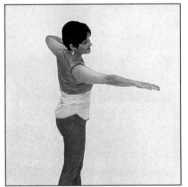

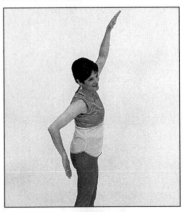

THE BACKSTROKE

"Smile every chance you get. People will smile back
and you will feel better for it."
—BETH, SIXTY-TWO

Pretend you're an Olympic gold medalist taking her celebratory lap in the pool.

STARTING POSITION: Stand with your feet hip-width apart. Place your arms straight in front of your body at shoulder height.

COUNTS: Every arm circle takes four counts.

STEP 1: Keeping your right arm as straight as possible, circle it back and down, and then return it to the starting position.

STEP 2: As your right arm is on its way down, begin making a similar backward circle with your left arm.

Make four circles with each arm.

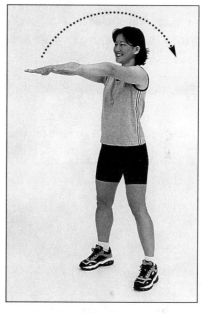

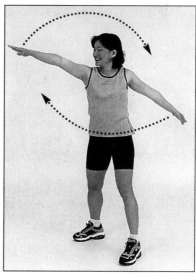

THE BREASTSTROKE

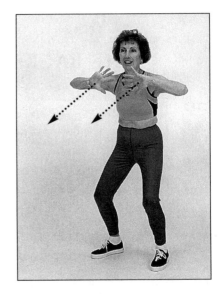

This exercise belongs to survivors—the *Breast*stroke! It is a chest expander and shoulder strengthener that also works the muscles between your shoulder blades.

STARTING POSITION: Stand with your feet hip-width apart and your knees slightly bent. Bring your hands together in front of your chest at shoulder height and let your elbows come up and out to the side. Your palms are facing front. Lean forward a tiny bit and look straight ahead.

COUNTS: Every Breaststroke takes four counts, or one count for each movement.

STEP 1: Push your palms forward, keeping them at shoulder height.

STEP 2: When your arms are fully extended in front of you, circle them out to your sides and simultaneously straighten your legs.

STEP 3: Keeping your legs straight, drop your arms to your sides. Then bend your knees and return to the starting position.
　　Repeat four times.

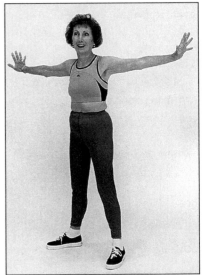

POINTERS:

◆ Be sure to spread your arms wide to the side to feel the expanse of the stretch across your chest.

◆ Inhale as you move your arms forward and exhale as you return them to the starting position.

OVERHEAD SIDE STRETCH

Whenever you stretch, it is incredibly useful to deepen your breathing because your muscles relax when they receive oxygen. You should feel this stretch along the sides of your rib cage.

STARTING POSITION: Stand with your feet hip-width apart; your arms hanging by your sides with the palms facing inward.

STEP 1: Swing your right arm slowly out to the side and up over your head. Your palm should be facing out. Gently tilt your body to the left and reach to the left with your right arm. Hold this position for two deep breaths in and out.

STEP 2: Return your body to an upright position and bring your right arm back down, making a slow, reaching arc.

Repeat the stretch on your left side.

Do two more stretches on each side.

POINTERS:

◆ Keep your palm facing outward even at the height of the stretch.

◆ Be gentle and move slowly.

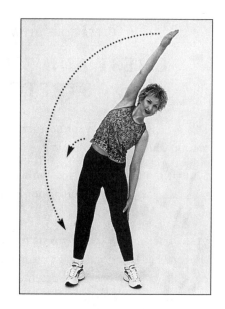

ARM ROCKING

Arm Rocking is slightly aerobic and increases your heart rate. It contains a series of arm movements at three different heights. The last two times you do the series you'll actually be moving around the room.

STARTING POSITION: Stand with your feet hip-width apart. Both arms are overhead in a giant C-shape. Your elbows are loose and the palms of your hands are facing each other.

COUNTS: Every arm rock is one count.

STEP 1: Maintaining the C-shape, rock your arms to the right. Then rock them back overhead and to the left.

STEP 2: Keeping the C-shape, lower your arms to shoulder height. Rock your arms to the right, and then rock them to the left.

STEP 3: Lower your arms in front of your thighs. Rock your arms to the right, as if you're ice-skating. Then rock them to the left. Again rock your arms to the right and left at this level.

STEP 4: Now walk around the room while you repeat the whole series.

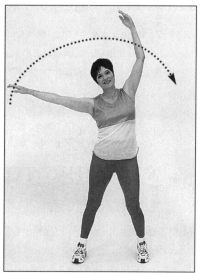

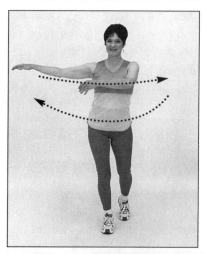

CHEST AND SHOULDER STRETCH

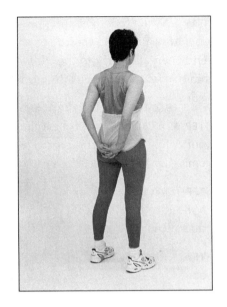

This exercise benefits your posture. It also stretches the tissue around your entire arm socket.

STARTING POSITION: Stand with your feet hip-width apart. Interlace your fingers behind your lower back with your palms facing up.

STEP 1: Straighten your arms as much as you can and inhale deeply while lifting your chest up and forward. Press your shoulders all the way back and down. Exaggerate the position by thinking about your shoulder blades coming together. Hold the position for two more deep breaths in and out.

STEP 2: Keeping your hands clasped, relax the position and slump your shoulders forward. Exhale.

Repeat the stretch four times.

CLIMBING THE LADDER

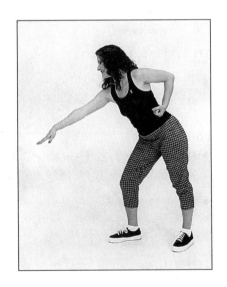

I recommend that you do this exercise slowly while you're learning to coordinate the movements. Once you get up to speed it's a lot of fun. Your weight is going to shift from side to side as you bend and straighten your right and left knees in turn. Your arms are going to move through a series of four positions—as though you were climbing up and down a ladder. The trick is to remember that at the same time your hands are alternately "climbing" up and then down, they are also pumping open and shut to increase your circulation.

STARTING POSITION: Stand with your feet hip-width apart. Make loose fists with your hands and place them at your waist.

COUNTS: Every movement takes two counts.

STEP 1: First, reach your right arm forward at waist height. Open your hand, bring your right shoulder forward, and bend your right knee, shifting your weight to your right leg.

STEP 2: Now reach your left arm forward at waist height, bend your left knee, bring your left shoulder forward, and open your left hand. Your weight shifts to your left leg. At the same time, straighten your right knee and pull your right hand back in to your waist, making a fist again.

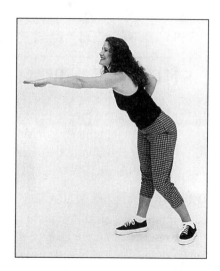

STEP 3: Reverse the arms, shoulders, and legs again—reaching your right hand forward to *shoulder height*, with your left hand coming back to your waist, where you make a fist.

STEP 4: Reverse the movements again. Reach your left arm out to *shoulder height* and pull your right hand back to your waist and make a fist.

STEP 5: Reverse the movements again. This time, though, reach your right arm forward to *face height*. Pull your left hand back to your waist.

STEP 6: Then do the reverse with your left arm to *face height* and your right arm coming into your waist.

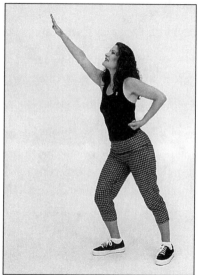

STEP 7: For the next four beats, alternate reaching *above your head* first with the right arm and then with the left arm, bending the same knee as the arm that is reaching upward. Continue opening your hand as your arm reaches full extension and closing your hand as it comes down to your shoulders.

STEP 8: Now repeat the same actions you made going up, this time moving downward. First reach your hands to *face height*, then reach them to *shoulder height*, and finally to *waist* height.
  Complete two whole series.

POINTERS:

◆ This series of movements must be performed slowly to protect you from injury.

◆ Imagine that you are squeezing two rubber balls as you open and close your fists.

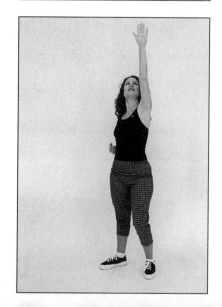

SHOULDER BLADE SQUEEZE

The Shoulder Blade Squeeze helps open your chest and shoulders as well as strengthen the muscles in your upper back. When you move your arms out to the sides you also get a good stretch along your entire arm.

STARTING POSITION: Stand with your feet hip-width apart. Bend your elbows and lift them to shoulder height so that your hands are in front of your chest, fingertips touching. Your palms are facing the floor. Your shoulders are dropped comfortably and even.

COUNTS: Each movement takes two counts.

STEP 1: Squeeze your shoulder blades together. Allow your fingertips to separate and your elbows to rotate behind you.

STEP 2: Return to the starting position. Repeat three times.

STEP 3: Now open your arms straight out to the sides keeping them at shoulder height and squeezing your shoulder blades together. Return to the starting position. Only do this movement once.

Repeat the entire series three times.

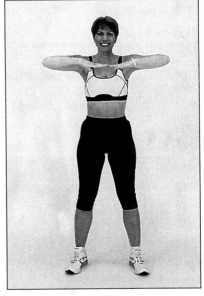

POINTERS:

◆ Keep your shoulders pressed lightly down.

◆ As you pull your elbows back, imagine your chest expanding gently forward.

◆ Stop whenever your arms feel fatigued. Do not overexert.

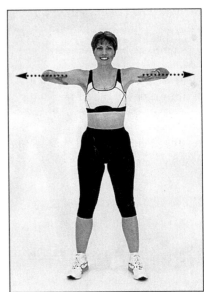

HEEL STRETCH

The Lower Body Ultimates are done seated in a chair without arms. Ideally your thighs should be parallel to the floor when your feet are flat. So try to use a chair that suits your height. This gives you stability and puts you into proper alignment. The Heel Stretch warms up the hamstring muscles located on the backs of the thighs.

STARTING POSITION: Sit on the front edge of your chair with both feet flat on the floor.

STEP 1: Extend your right leg forward and rest it on the heel. Flex your right foot.

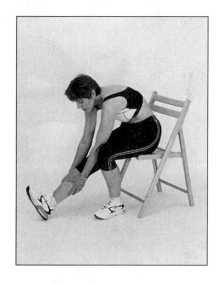

STEP 2: Keeping your leg as straight as possible and your spine straight, bend forward from the hips and reach out to your right shin with both hands. Hold this position and breathe deeply into the stretch for at least eight counts. Take your time. This is a long, slow stretch. Return your leg to the starting position.

Repeat the stretch with your left leg.

POINTERS:

◆ Breathe and relax. This enables your hamstring to soften and stretch farther. You may notice that your stretch deepens as you stay in it.

◆ Don't force yourself forward. Just go to the edge of your ability and hold there.

◆ Because you're seated on the edge of the chair, remember to keep most of your weight back on the chair rather than forward over your leg. From time to time, I've seen women fall off their chairs doing this stretch. Please don't risk it.

SINGLE AND DOUBLE LEG LIFTS

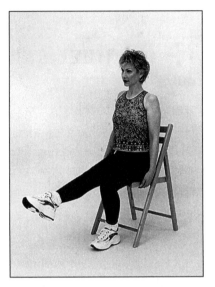

Concentrating on your quadriceps, the muscles located on the front of your thighs, can help you reap the benefits of this simple exercise, which uses several muscle groups.

STARTING POSITION: Sit all the way back in your chair, but remain upright instead of leaning back. Your feet should be flat on the floor, your spine straight, and your shoulders lightly pressed down. Think about pulling your tummy in, while you keep breathing.

COUNTS: Every movement takes two counts.

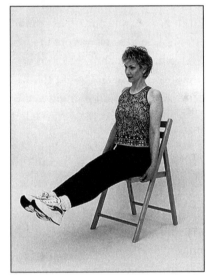

STEP 1: Straighten your right leg in front of you and point your toes. Hold for two counts. Then lower it to the starting position and relax your foot. Do eight Single Leg Lifts.

Repeat with your left leg.

STEP 2: Next, straighten both legs in front of you, pointing the toes. Hold for two counts. As you lower your legs to the starting position relax your feet. Do eight Double Leg Lifts.

POINTERS:

◆ For extra stability you may hold on to the sides of the chair. Use your arms to give you some leverage as you lift your legs.

◆ Holding your stomach will help you remain upright.

◆ Move slowly through the repetitions. It's a simple exercise but it has many benefits.

FOOT FLEX

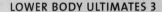

"Take one day at a time. Don't wish your life away."
—MARIE, FIFTY-FIVE

The Foot Flex is a simple yet important exercise. Having strong and flexible feet and ankles is the foundation of balance.

STARTING POSITION: Sit back in your chair with your feet flat on the floor, your spine erect, your shoulders down and back, and your tummy lifted.

COUNTS: Each flex or point takes one count.

STEP 1: Straighten your right leg so that it's parallel to the floor. In this position, first flex your foot, and then point your foot. Flex and point your right foot four times. Then lower your leg.
   Repeat with your left leg and foot.

STEP 2: Now straighten both legs and point and flex both feet eight times.

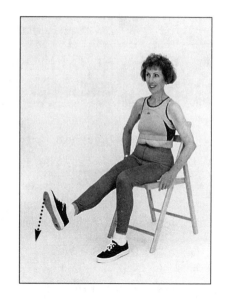

LEG SCISSORS

Leg Scissors work the muscles of your inner and outer thighs. Focusing your attention on these target areas as you move increases the benefits you receive.

STARTING POSITION: Sit back in your chair. Check your posture. Lift both legs straight in front of you, and point your toes.

COUNTS: Each movement takes two counts.

STEP 1: Open your legs to the side to a distance of two feet. Then bring them back together with your right leg over the left.

STEP 2: Open your legs again. This time, as you bring them back together, bring your left leg over your right.
   Scissor like this eight times.

POINTERS:

◆ Hold on to the sides of the chair for support.

◆ Pull your stomach muscles in strongly as you do these moves.

◆ You don't need to bring your legs very wide apart to get the full benefit of this exercise.

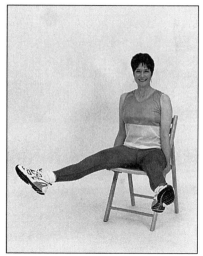

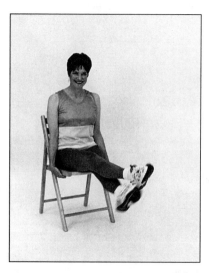

ONE-LEGGED BUTTERFLY

This exercise may seem a little weird at first. People with tight hips often find it extremely challenging. It is, however, extremely beneficial. Over time it can open up your whole hip socket, your lower back, and your lower abdominal muscles.

STARTING POSITION: Sit on the edge of your chair or back in your chair, whichever feels most comfortable. Your feet are hip-width apart and flat on the floor. Hold on to the edges of your seat for stability.

STEP 1: Bring your right foot up and cross your ankle over your left knee. Let your right knee fall open to the side.

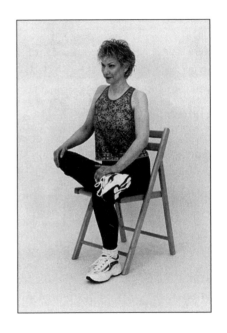

STEP 2: Place your left hand on your right ankle. With your right hand, gently press down on your right knee. Hold for several long, slow counts. Breathe deeply into the stretch. Then lower your right foot to the starting position.

Do the same stretch with your left leg.

Repeat the set.

POINTERS:

◆ Stay relaxed and do not force the stretch.

◆ Remember to breathe in deeply through your nose and exhale through your mouth.

STOMACH CONTRACTIONS

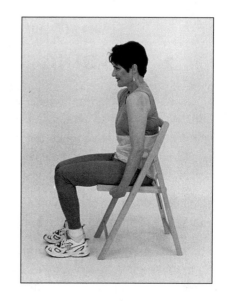

I first learned about this exercise years ago by reading a magazine interview with a movie star. She claimed it was the reason her stomach was as flat as a board. Well, if movie stars can do it, we certainly can. Hollywood has nothing on us!

STARTING POSITION: Sit in your chair with your feet hip-width apart and flat on the floor. Check your posture.

COUNTS: Each Stomach Contraction takes four counts.

STEP 1: Pull your stomach back to meet your spine, while allowing your buttocks to roll slightly forward under you. Your shoulders should also round slightly forward. Imagine you are trying to get into a tight pair of jeans and the zipper is stuck. Exhale as you suck your stomach in.

STEP 2: Then release and inhale.

Contract four times. As you get stronger, work up to eight repetitions.

DERRIERE ISOMETRICS

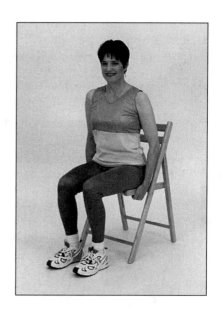

La belle derriere! (That's a fancy way of saying "Your beautiful butt.") The point of this exercise is to tone and tighten your backside.

STARTING POSITION: Sit in your chair with your legs hip-width apart and feet flat on the floor. Your arms should hang by your sides.

COUNTS: Each Derriere Isometric takes four counts.

STEP 1: Squeeze your butt muscles together as hard as you possibly can. Hold for two slow breaths in and out. Release. Then rest for two more slow breaths.

Squeeze eight times.

HANGING SPIRALS

This exercise is one of my all-time favorites since it makes my back feel so good. It literally creates space between each of your vertebra, releasing pressure on the nerves and improving your circulation. In addition, this seated exercise increases the circulation in your arms, arm sockets, and shoulders.

STARTING POSITION: Sit all the way back in your chair with your knees close together and your feet flat on the floor.

STEP 1: Roll your upper body slowly forward, until your head and arms are dangling toward your feet, as though you were trying to recover from a faint. First, bend your head forward until your chin touches your chest. Then let your shoulders cave in. Then the rest of the spine starts rounding down, one vertebra at a time. Hold at the bottom, bending forward at the hips and leaning your chest against your thighs. Your arms and head are dangling forward.

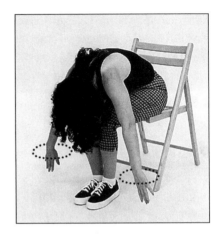

STEP 2: Now make small circles above the floor with both your hands, four times in one direction and then four times in the opposite direction. Repeat.

STEP 3: Slowly roll up through your spine. As you come up, bring your arms up in front of your body and then overhead.

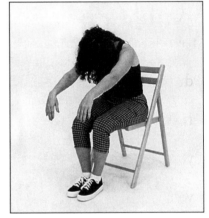

STEP 4: Flex your wrists so that your palms are facing the ceiling and your fingertips are pointing inward. Keeping your wrists flexed, slowly lower your arms out to the sides and then down. Relax.

POINTERS:

◆ You may feel fluid rushing into your hands. This is normal.

◆ If you have any difficulty rolling up, feel free to put your hands on your thighs and give yourself a little leverage.

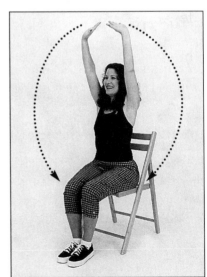

BUILDING STRENGTH

When you have achieved complete range of motion and feel no pain during the Upper Body Ultimates, you may choose to add this set of isometric strengthening exercises to your workout. Isometrics can be a safer way for you, as a survivor, to build muscular strength on your own than using free weights or weight machines. If you do choose to weight train, please get professional direction from a trainer who is familiar with the ramifications of breast cancer surgery and lymphedema.

Isometric exercises target individual muscles rather than groups of muscles. Thus you know and can feel precisely what is being worked during a given exercise. When you focus your attention on a muscle, it responds by growing stronger more quickly. By keeping your movements slow during isometrics, the physical sensations will tell you if something is going wrong so that you'll know if you need to stop.

Before doing the Building Strength exercises, always be sure to warm up with the Basic Warm-up and the Upper Body Ultimates. You don't want to do these exercises cold or prior to stretching your body. It is not recommended to do this section on its own, although you may omit the Lower Body Ultimates on those occasions when you need to shorten your workout time. These can be done properly either seated or standing.

WHAT YOU NEED FOR BUILDING STRENGTH
You'll need an elastic exercise band. Choose one without handles, such as a Dynaband or Theraband. You'll need to grasp it at various points of length during your workout, sometimes placing your hands closer and sometimes farther apart. Bands with handles don't give you this option.

Elastic bands come in different colors that indicate various levels of resistance. Resistance is what takes the place of a heavy weight in these exercises. I recommend that you start off with the least resistant band and then gradually build up to using the more resistant ones. As you get stronger and more flexible, moving your hands closer together can further increase the resistance of your band.

Since they give you more options and greater control, elastic bands are ideal for someone who must be especially sensitive to her body. When you use a band, you are constantly in control of the degree of pressure under which your muscles are working. In addition, the minute you feel any pain or fatigue you can simply let go.

There were two survivors in one of my classes who had arthritis and so weren't able to grip their elastic bands in a fist. But we found a good solution. We slotted the band between their thumbs and palms at a loose resistance. As a result, they were able to enjoy every exercise in this section.

Store your band at room temperature. Rubber can soften and lose its shape when heated or crack when it gets too cold. Elastic bands are made of the same kind of thin, floppy material that a dentist uses to build a dental dam, so they are susceptible. The moment you see striated lines in your band, replace it. That means it is losing its integrity. Bands generally last for about six months with repeated use.

Caution: After breast surgery there is always a risk of developing lymphedema. As a survivor, you never want to wrap an elastic band around your hand and impede your circulation in any way. This is vital to your safety and continued good health. Therefore always let the ends of your workout band dangle freely.

SHOULDER BLADE CONTRACTION

The outward and inward movements of the Shoulder Blade Contraction are equally important. You are using two different sets of muscles to perform each.

STARTING POSITION: Stand or sit with your feet hip-width apart. Check your posture. Hold the band in a loose overhanded grip near your chest. Your hands are about a foot and a half apart. Your elbows are lifted to shoulder height.

COUNTS: Four counts to extend and four counts to return.

STEP 1: Straighten your arms slowly out to the sides. Feel your shoulder blades pull together and your chest expand forward.

STEP 2: Then, slowly bend your elbows and return your hands to the starting position.

   Repeat four times. You may build up to six when you feel strong enough and in complete control.

POINTERS:

◆ Don't arch your back.

◆ Resist the elastic band as you slowly return.

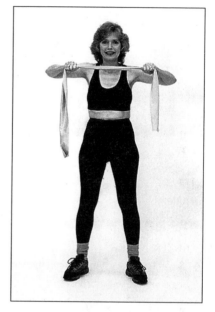

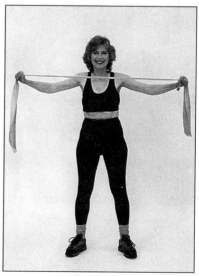

YAWN STRETCH

You know how wonderful it can feel when you get up first thing in the morning and take that delicious initial stretch? That is what this exercise is like. It always makes me feel extra good.

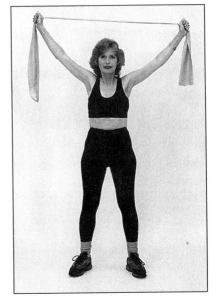

STARTING POSITION: Sit or stand with your feet hip-width apart. Extend your arms over your head and hold your elastic band in an overhanded grip. Your hands are spread about a foot and a half apart. Keep your elbows straight.

COUNTS: Four counts down and four counts up.

STEP 1: Spread your arms open and back as far as you can, as if you are having a huge yawn. Keep your arms straight and bring your hands as close to shoulder level as possible. Inhale deeply. The band should run behind your head, if possible.

STEP 2: Then bring your hands back up to the starting position. Exhale.

Do four times. Work up to six repetitions when you are able.

POINTER:

◆ Watch out for your hair. When it gets caught in the band it can be a nightmare to untangle. The best thing is to tie your hair back in a ponytail.

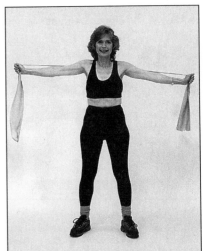

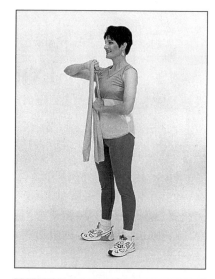

OUTER AND INNER ARM PULL

"I have improved my strength and muscle tone so much by using the Building Strength exercises that I have gone from the weakest color band to the strongest color band. I love the way my upper body looks and feels."

—DIANE, FIFTY-FOUR

STARTING POSITION: Sit or stand with your feet hip-width apart. Bring your hands to touch your breastbone so that they are stacked, the right above the left. The left hand is facing toward your body and the right is facing out from your body. Each hand grips the elastic band, with a distance of six inches to one foot between them. When the right arm is working, the left hand anchors the band in place and vice versa.

COUNTS: Every movement takes two counts.

STEP 1: Push your right hand up above your head until your elbow is straight. Allow your head to follow your hand, so that at the top of the movement you are gazing upward. Bring your right hand and head back to the starting position.

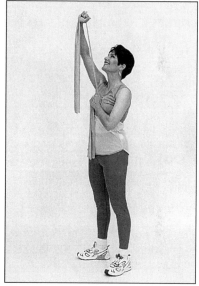

STEP 2: Now straighten your right arm out to the side. Turn your head to the right to follow your hand. Return your arm and head to the starting position.

STEP 3: Repeat the series with your left arm.
   Do two more sets on the right and left.

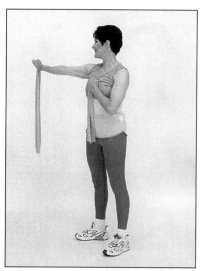

CHEST EXPANDER

The Chest Expander is an efficient series of movements that can truly increase your power and endurance when you commit to doing it regularly.

STARTING POSITION: Place the elastic band around your back where your bra strap goes, as if you are measuring your bust line with a measuring tape. Hold the band in an overhanded grip with your hands directly in front of your armpits. Make sure the band is on the outside of your arms. The ends should dangle from your thumbs not your little fingers.

COUNTS: Every movement takes two counts.

STEP 1: Push your hands directly forward until your elbows are straight.

STEP 2: Then let the band pull your straight arms out to the sides and back, expanding your chest. Breathe in deeply.

STEP 3: Reverse directions by pulling your straight arms back to the front. Then bring your hands back to your armpits.
Repeat. Build up to four repetitions, as you get stronger.

POINTERS:

♦ You will probably need to experiment with how much slack you need on your band in order to reach the full extension forward.

♦ Do not allow the band to touch any part of your arms when they are open to the sides.

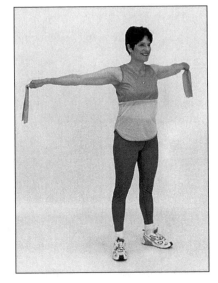

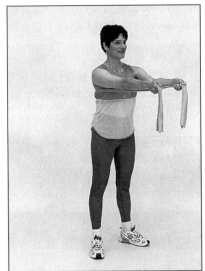

BICEP CURL

The Bicep Curl targets the muscles of your chest near the armpit and the upper and lower parts of your arms. To get the full benefits of the movement, concentrate on tightening your bicep muscle as you do it.

STARTING POSITION: Step on one end of your band, either with the heel or the ball of your right foot. Hold the other end of the band in your right hand. The palm of your hand is turned forward, and the end of your band dangles from the little finger side of your fist. Lock your right arm tight against the side of your body. Your wrist should be straight, not flexed during this exercise and you should stand tall.

COUNTS: Four counts to curl and four counts to release.

STEP 1: Bend your right elbow and slowly bring your hand up to your shoulder. Return slowly to the starting position. Repeat four times.

STEP 2: Switch the elastic band to your left hand and foot. When you are ready, repeat the Bicep Curl four times with your left arm.

POINTER:

◆ I find that I have more balance and strength when I put the foot on my working side a little bit behind the other. But this is a matter of preference. You should take the stance that is most comfortable for you.

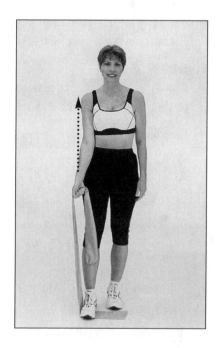

ROWING

Rowing is a strengthener for the triceps muscles on the outside of your upper arm (an area most women would like to see looking more toned and sculpted). Do not rush the movements, the effort of resisting as you release is as important as pulling upward.

STARTING POSITION: Step on one end of your elastic band with your right foot. Grip the other end of the band in your right hand. Let it dangle from the little finger side of your fist. Your

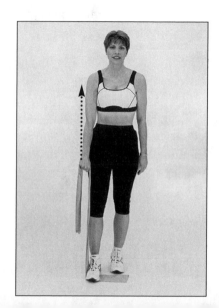

right arm is by your side with the palm of your right hand facing backward.

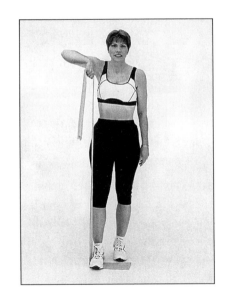

COUNTS: Every movement takes two counts.

STEP 1: Keeping your right hand close to the side of your body, pull your right elbow out to the side and up to shoulder height. Then return your arm to the starting position.

Repeat four times. Build up to six repetitions, as you are able.

STEP 2: Switch the elastic band to your left foot and left hand. Repeat four times with your left arm.

POINTERS:

◆ Find a comfortable foot position, one that is stable and gives you your preferred amount of resistance.

◆ Keep your wrists straight, rather than flexed.

BUILDING STRENGTH 7

BIG HUG

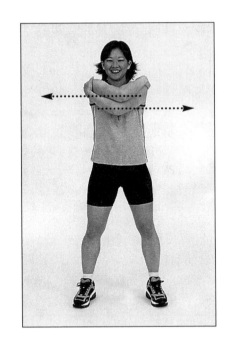

Who loves you, baby? You do. Now you deserve a little affection.

STARTING POSITION: Drop your workout band. Extend your arms out to your sides at shoulder height.

COUNTS: Take your sweet time.

STEP 1: Wrap your arms around yourself in a Big Hug with your right arm on top.

STEP 2: Extend your arms to the sides again. Then hug yourself with your left arm on top.

Congratulations! You have finished the Upper and Lower Ultimates as well as the Building Strength exercises. Now please continue with the Ultimate Dance Routine and Healing Visualization that follow.

THE ULTIMATE DANCE ROUTINE

Here is the most fun part of the program. Put on your favorite dance number and get ready to move. The Ultimate Dance Routine is designed to last about five minutes. Enjoy yourself and don't worry about making mistakes. This is your time to let go and express yourself.

Since you have now achieved a full range of motion without pain (the only requirements for using the Ultimate Movements), feel free on occasion to substitute one of the additional dance routines in the book for variety. These appear after each of the exercise programs in Part Two, "Adjusting to the Needs of Your New Body."

MUSICAL SUGGESTION: "Shackles" by Mary Mary from the album *Thankful*.

STARTING POSITION: Stand with your feet together. Your hands are flexed toward the ceiling at your shoulders. Fingertips point backward.

COUNTS: Every movement takes one count.

STEP-TOGETHER-STEP-TOUCH: You're going to travel right. Step out and shift your weight onto your right foot. Step your left foot beside it. Step out again onto your right foot. Touch your left foot beside the right without placing your weight on it. As you touch, push your hands straight up.

Bring your hands back to shoulder height as you begin to travel left, stepping out with your left foot. Do the same series in reverse: step-together-step-touch. Push your hands to the ceiling as you touch your right foot.

Do four sets. Then go on to Step Kicks.

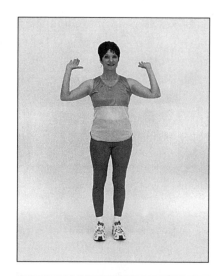

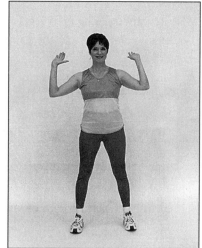

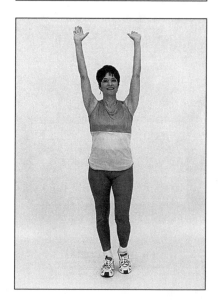

STEP KICKS: Step onto your right foot and kick your left leg to the right. Then step onto your left foot and kick your right leg to the left. Clap your hands when you kick.

Repeat eight times. Then go on to Arm Rocking.

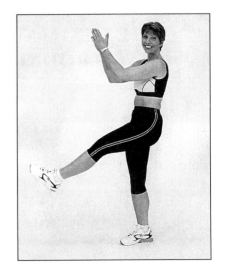

ARM ROCKING: Bring both arms overhead in a giant C-shape. Your elbows are loose and the palms of your hands are facing each other.

Walk around the room as you rock your arms to the right, then rock them back overhead and to the left.

Lower your arms to chest height. Keeping the C-shape, rock your arms to the right, then rock them to the left.

Lower your arms in front of your thighs. Rock your arms to the right, as if you're ice-skating. Then rock them to the left. Repeat at this height.

Repeat the whole set of arm rocks. Then go on to Reach for the Stars.

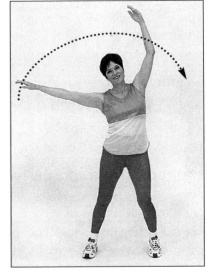

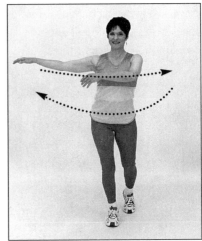

REACH FOR THE STARS: Reach your right arm up, as though you are trying to touch a star. Then reach farther for a second count. Bring your right hand down to your hip.

Now reach up the same way with your left arm.

Do four sets.

Keep on repeating the whole routine from beginning to end until the song ends. Then take a slow walk around the room, or walk in place, to lower your heart rate and cool down. Breathe deeply in and out to supply your body with the oxygen it needs. Have a refreshing drink of water.

Spend a few quiet moments doing the Healing Visualization that follows.

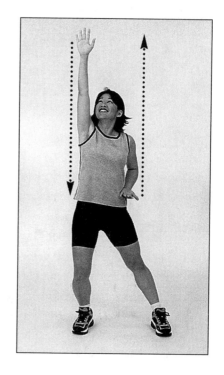

HEALING VISUALIZATION
FOR THRIVERS

Sit in a chair in a comfortable position with your feet flat on the floor and your spine erect and supported. Close your eyes. Breathe deeply in through your nose and out through your mouth. You are going to take this opportunity to get in touch with yourself on many levels of your being.

First, scan your physical body from head to toe. Are you holding any tension? See if you can let it go. Imagine that you are being filled with golden light as if from a pitcher of warm water that is pouring into you. When the liquid relaxation reaches the crown of your head, it overflows and cascades all around you, surrounding you in a bubble of light. Ask your physical body if there is anything it needs from you. See if there is one word that would describe your physical being right now.

Now scan your emotional body. What emotions are you feeling right now? Do they register in any particular area of your body? Can you embrace your feelings instead of resist them? Ask your emotional body what it needs. See if there is a message for you. Is there one word that would best describe your emotional state?

Next, check in with your mental being. Are your thoughts active or still right now? Are you holding on to judgments or concerns or is your mind clear?

Acknowledge how your mind serves you. Thank it for helping you. Ask your mind if there is anything it needs from you right now. See if there is one word that would describe your mental state.

Can you slip into the space between your thoughts? For a moment or more, can you transcend your body, emotions, and mind?

Attune yourself to your spiritual being. Connect to your heart and your soul. Would you like to offer up a prayer or a request for guidance? Is there anyone for whom or anything for which you feel especially grateful or loving? Sit with that. Allow your love and gratitude to magnify and expand.

Visualize something beautiful: a place, a person, an experience that makes you feel fulfilled, relaxed, joyful, or in awe. Perhaps it is a flower. Hold that image for as long as you would like.

Finally, say to yourself three times, "Today I'm alive, and I'm going to live as well as I can!" whatever that means to you.

When you feel ready, open your eyes, and come back to the room.

On other occasions, for a little variety, you may practice the healing visualizations in Part Two, "Adjusting to the Needs of Your New Body."

PART FOUR

Sports Warm-ups

Participation in sports can be one of the best ways to restore confidence in your capabilities and make peace with your body after breast cancer. It can elevate your spirits tremendously. Sports draw upon your competitive spirit, personal image, and expand your sense of what is possible. As you have already seen by working on the routines in the earlier sections of this book, exercise is an integral part of the healing process. In addition, sports are fun and a great opportunity to connect and socialize with people.

Whether you have been active or inactive in the past, there is absolutely no reason why, as a survivor, you can't participate in sports today. The most you need to do is take appropriate precautions, get enough rest after participating, and pay attention to the signals your body sends you. Remind yourself that it may take some time to get back up to speed, so give yourself permission to progress in stages. Long-term survivors generally know their limitations, but may surprise themselves. Your body, your mind, and your spirit all hold amazing unrealized potentials that can be accessed through sports.

It is perfectly appropriate and wise, if you so choose, to seek the advice of professional sports trainers with expertise in helping breast cancer survivors. While certifications vary from sport to sport, you can always ask your trainer to sit down with you and your physician to discuss your unique circumstances and needs. Think of this as an educational process for you and for them. To find a trainer, you may ask for a referral from your oncologist or surgeon. Also try contacting the American College of Sports Medicine (see Resources). Be proactive. Ask around and interview personal trainers at gyms and health clubs until you find the one who makes you feel most comfortable.

I have put together this section of sport-specific warm-ups to assist you in safely continuing to pursue the activities you love. Each program begins with the Basic Warm-up and then varies according to the muscles that the particular sport targets and any challenges it might hold for survivors. Both the assets and the drawbacks of the sport are briefly outlined. Please show these specifics to your trainer and/or physician and discuss them.

In my opinion, you should only undertake these sports after you've mastered the Ultimate Movements. If you have physical issues, such as pain, loss of range of motion, and unsteady balance, among others, I would also suggest that you turn back to Part Two, "Adjusting to the Needs of Your New Body," for guidance. Otherwise, feel free to move on to the warm-up routine for your sport and begin.

Have fun!

WALKING

"Keep a positive attitude. After all, what's your alternative?"

—Diane, fifty-three

$\mathcal{D}$iane had a family history of breast cancer, so she was always careful to go for an annual checkup. Her mammogram in March 1999 came back "clean." That autumn, however, in the fitting room of the store where she was shopping for a bra to match a new party dress, she found a lump in her breast. It felt more like a gummy bear than the pea-sized lump that she had been told to hunt for in self-exams. Diane panicked and called a doctor friend, and went for a mammogram and a sonogram that very day.

Because of her family history, Diane opted for a double mastectomy with reconstruction. After the first surgery, she had so much skin left over that she felt like one of those wrinkled dogs called a shar-pei. Two weeks later, in a second surgery, her doctor put chest expanders into the muscles of her chest wall, which left her incredibly sore. Her final outpatient procedure was the insertion of saline implants. During the three weeks it took her to heal from this, her breasts felt so heavy with all the fluid that her husband literally had to help her sit up in order to get out of bed. The tenderness was so great and she felt so short of breath that it took her five months to get back to walking. Prior to surgery she had been an active walker and she missed her daily excursions.

Now, walking more than a short distance would bring on horrible cramps in Diane's calves, thighs, and arches. So for homework outside class, I gave her a series of exercises to build the strength in her legs. She began stretching diligently before and after walking. Soon the cramps were history. But she also had to relearn how to balance, since the weight of her implants was greater than her own breasts had been. Doing Focus on Healing three times a week and taking daily walking excursions substantially improved her equilibrium.

Today, nothing stops Diane from walking. She is an interior designer who finds considerable beauty in architecture and landscapes, and as she takes her morning walk through different neighborhoods she observes the details of the houses, windows, fences, and yards searching for new ideas. It gives her mind a creative workout at the same time her body is getting stronger. Diane has a positive attitude, a good sense of humor, and feels grateful for the tremendous love and support of her family and friends. Although her balance is not yet perfect, two years after reconstruc-

tion, it is much better and no longer interferes with her keeping busy and living life.

WALKING SPECIFICS FOR SURVIVORS Walking is wonderful cardiovascular exercise. It mostly targets the muscles in your lower body—the abdomen, buttocks, and legs. You can also target your biceps and triceps muscles by pumping your arms.

As a survivor, it is important, while walking, to raise your arms above your head from time to time to keep the fluid from pooling in them, especially if you are at risk for lymphedema. But there is nothing to stop you from walking as soon as you get home from the hospital and for the rest of your life.

THE WARM-UP:

◆ The Basic Warm-up (pp. 15–23)
◆ Mountain High Stretch
◆ The Crawl
◆ The Backstroke

MOUNTAIN HIGH STRETCH

Begin here, after doing the Basic Warm-up. Do this stretch before walking.

STARTING POSITION: Stand with your feet hip-width apart, your arms hanging by your sides.

STEP 1: Bring both arms forward and up, until they are overhead. Hook your fingers together and turn the palms of your hands up to the ceiling. Pull your shoulders up toward your ears. Inhale as you stretch up.

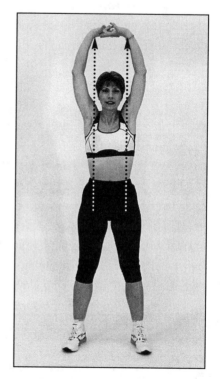

STEP 2: Keeping your fingers interlaced, press your shoulders down hard. Exhale.

Repeat steps 1 and 2 four times.

STEP 3: Next, still keeping your fingers interlaced, tilt your body to the right. Hold and breathe deeply.

STEP 4: Come upright again and tilt to the left. Hold and breathe deeply.

STEP 5: Come upright again and unhook your fingers. With your wrists flexed, slowly lower your arms out to the sides and return them to the starting position.

Do two complete sets.

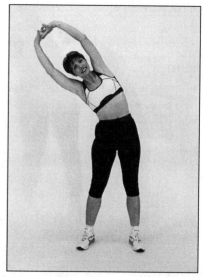

POINTER:

◆ Keep your elbows as straight as possible when your fingers are interlocked.

THE CRAWL

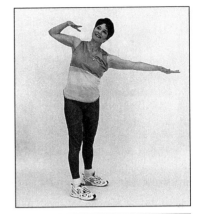

You can do the Crawl as you walk to get your circulation going and stretch out your shoulders.

STARTING POSITION: Stand with your feet hip-width apart. Your arms should be straight out in front of your body at shoulder height—or as high as you can lift them.

COUNTS: Every arm circle takes eight counts.

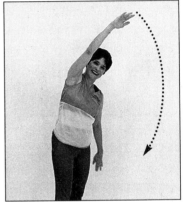

STEP 1: To do the Crawl, your arms must cycle independently. Lower your right arm down to your side, then bend your right elbow and bring the arm up to shoulder height. From shoulder height, continue the movement by extending the arm straight up in the air.

STEP 2: At the same time, bring your left arm down to your side, then bend the left elbow and bring your left arm up to shoulder height. As the left arm is rising, circle the right arm forward and down to the starting position. As the left arm continues straight up into the air, lower your right arm to your side.

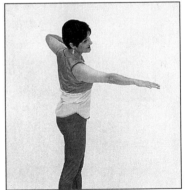

Circle both arms four times. Turn your head to the right as your right hand reaches your shoulder and then turn it to the left as your left hand reaches your shoulder. Your movements are continuous and flowing. Try to find a steady rhythm.

POINTER:

◆ Imagine the resistance of the water.

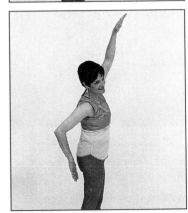

THE BACKSTROKE

While you are walking, occasionally do the Backstroke to increase your range of motion and improve your circulation.

STARTING POSITION: Stand with your feet hip-width apart. Place your arms straight in front of your body at shoulder height.

COUNTS: Every arm circle takes four counts.

STEP 1: Keeping your right arm as straight as possible, circle it back and down, and then return it to the starting position.

STEP 2: As your right arm is on its way down, begin making a similar backward circle with your left arm.
 Make four circles with each arm.

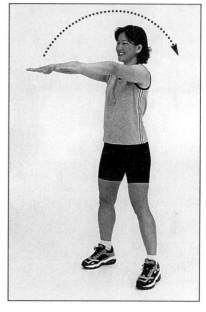

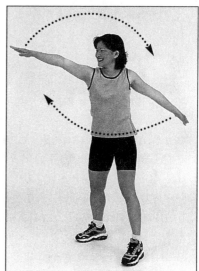

RUNNING

"I have been through so much, but, yes, I am through it. I am alive today. I am well today. I try to live each day with a purpose—not a grand purpose, just a purpose."

—*Susan, fifty-six*

For nearly twenty-five years, Susan has been a runner. When her kids were little, she ran every day and enjoyed excellent health. Then, at thirty-five, she found a lump in her right breast during a self-examination and underwent a lumpectomy and radiation. As soon as she could she started running again. Once she was past the five-year mark she was sure she had licked cancer for good. Working part-time, she raised two children as a single parent and kept up her exercise. She spent seventeen years cancer-free.

In 1996, she was diagnosed with another cancer in the same breast. This time she had a mastectomy. While she was doing a course of outpatient chemotherapy she walked to maintain her stamina. She was too fatigued to run, and could barely make it around the block. It was a rough time. After a few months going around a track, she started gentle jogging. At one point her blood counts dropped and she had to ease up on her program. But she worked her way back and, by alternating running and walking at first, finally built up her distance to three miles.

Two years later she had another recurrence with invaded lymph nodes. She had another surgery, more radiation, and a stem cell transplant. Now Susan has lymphedema and has to watch her heart rate when she runs so that she won't overload her lymphatic system. She gets tired more easily and sometimes her feet feel numb. Nonetheless, through it all, she keeps on running.

When Susan runs she can feel her whole body working in unison. Her mind and body are free. It is an effortless, fluid motion. She finds it to be a terrific antidepressant. Her symptoms sometimes slow her down, but they haven't made her quit yet. Running is the best way Susan knows to achieve inner peace and a sense of health and wholeness.

RUNNING SPECIFICS FOR SURVIVORS For the most part running works the muscles of your lower body, your abdomen, buttocks, and legs. It is a great exercise for the heart and lungs. If you have never run before, take it slow at first, alternating walking and running short distances. Build up slowly about 10 percent more distance each week. Make sure to do the Basic Warm-up and warm up your shoulders, chest, and arms.

The only reason for caution is the risk of lymphedema. Pumping your arms and elevating your heart rate can sometimes trigger symptoms. Reread the Eighteen Steps to Prevent Lymphedema (p. 6). Overexertion can cause the lymphatic system to back up and your arm to swell. So get your stretches in and be sure to raise your arms overhead from time to time when you are running (to determine your target heart rate see p. 8). Listen to the signals your body sends you about what it needs—you are probably exercising too hard if your heart is pounding and you are short of breath.

THE WARM-UP
- The Basic Warm-up (pp. 15–23)
- Mountain High Stretch
- Overhead Side Stretch
- Around the World

MOUNTAIN HIGH STRETCH

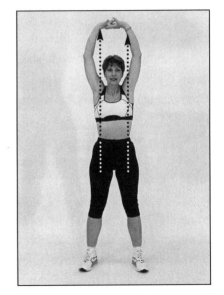

Begin here, after doing the Basic Warm-up.

STARTING POSITION: Stand with your feet hip-width apart, your arms hanging by your sides.

STEP 1: Bring both arms forward and up, until they are overhead. Hook your fingers together and turn the palms of your hands up to the ceiling. Pull your shoulders up toward your ears. Inhale as you stretch up.

STEP 2: Keeping your fingers interlaced, press your shoulders down hard. Exhale.

Repeat steps 1 and 2 four times.

STEP 3: Next, still keeping your fingers interlaced, tilt your body to the right. Hold and breathe deeply.

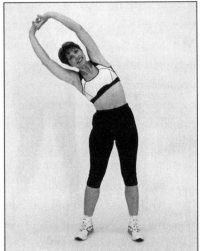

STEP 4: Come upright again and tilt to the left. Hold and breathe deeply.

STEP 5: Come upright again and unhook your fingers. With your wrists flexed, slowly lower your arms out to the sides and return them to the starting position.

Do two complete sets.

POINTER:

◆ Keep your elbows as straight as possible when your fingers are interlocked.

OVERHEAD SIDE STRETCH

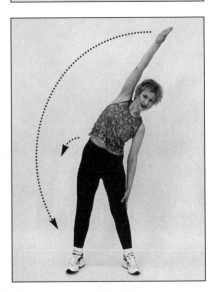

STARTING POSITION: Stand with you feet hip-width apart; your arms hanging by your sides with the palms facing inward.

STEP 1: Swing your right arm slowly out to the side and up over your head. Your palm should be facing out. Gently tilt your body to the left and reach to the left with your right arm. Hold this position for two deep breaths in and out.

STEP 2: Return your body to an upright position and bring your right arm back down, making a slow, reaching arc.

Repeat the stretch on your left side.

Do two more stretches on each side.

POINTERS:

◆ Keep your palm facing outward even at the height of the stretch.

◆ Be gentle and move slowly.

RUNNING 3

AROUND THE WORLD

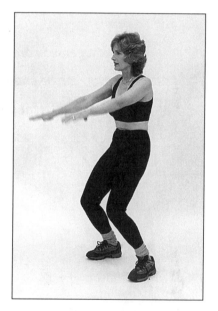

STARTING POSITION: Stand with your feet hip-width apart, your arms hanging by your sides.

COUNTS: A complete circle takes four counts.

STEP 1: Bend your knees as you raise your arms forward and overhead.

STEP 2: Straighten your knees as you circle your arms backward and then down to the starting position. Repeat.

STEP 3: Now reverse the circle, bending your knees while bringing your arms back and up behind your head.

STEP 4: Straighten your knees as you circle your arms forward and down to the starting position. Repeat.

POINTERS:

◆ The knee bend at the beginning of the movement should feel as if you were about to spring lightly off a diving board.

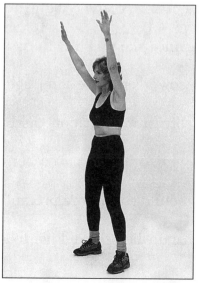

SWIMMING

*"When you are diagnosed with cancer, your perceptions of
who you can be and what you can do opens up. Allow yourself to see
the different parts of yourself. You can reinvent yourself
and try to do anything you want."*

—Karen, thirty-seven

*K*aren might not have discovered her cancer as soon as she did
since she was just thirty years old—younger than average. But a friend and
coworker of the same age was diagnosed with cancer, so she decided to do a
breast examination right away. Her breasts felt lumpy, which was nothing
new. Still, she asked her doctor for a mammogram and then had an ultrasound as an extra precaution. They asked her to come back six months later,
and when she did her follow-up ultrasound showed some changes. A biopsy

then revealed cancer. Karen's immediate reaction was disbelief. "Not me!" What were the odds of two young coworkers both getting cancer at the same time? But it was true. For treatment, she underwent a lumpectomy, node dissection, and radiation therapy.

Karen had been a swimmer for many years before her diagnosis, but during her radiation treatment she was not allowed to swim. Instead, she cross-trained by walking and jogging. The radiation wore her out so much that she still felt fatigued six weeks after her treatment ended. By then she was back in the pool slowly working to rebuild her fitness level. One day she noticed that she was tired in the old familiar way, not in the way she felt from radiation. It was a turning point, a moment of restoration and healing. She felt in control of her body once again.

Today, Karen is a director of a group called Team Survivors in California. She got involved because she believes that athletic activity after cancer teaches you about your capabilities. She finds the weightlessness in water to be a wonderfully therapeutic sensation—a feeling shared by many survivors who experience weight gain from treatment. She especially loves how graceful she feels in the water, even though she doesn't necessarily feel that way on land. She also knows that swimming is an excellent means of stretching scar tissue and muscles.

SWIMMING SPECIFICS FOR SURVIVORS Swimming is one of the very best activities for breast cancer survivors. It works all your muscles from head to toe, and swim strokes help increase your range of motion and decrease your pain. It is a perfect complement to the Focus on Healing program. It is a good idea to consult a knowledgeable aquatic trainer for assistance in designing an appropriate personal swimming program.

There is something exceptionally restorative about being submersed in water. In water you may feel as though your troubles are simply washing away. Water has two other wonderful qualities. It supports you against gravity, so you feel weightless, and there is little impact for sore muscles and joints. In addition, the harder you push against water, the more resistance you create to your own movement. Therefore you can easily control the degree of your effort and the difficulty of your workout.

If you are still in treatment of any kind speak with your doctors about swimming before you begin or resume it. The advice you receive may depend on your stage of recovery or treatment. For instance, when I was in radiation my radiologist did not want me in a pool that contained chlorine. There can be many issues to be considered, such as immunity and skin irritation. Your radiologist can help you assess when it is okay for you to start swimming again.

THE WARM-UP
- The Basic Warm-up (pp. 15–23)
- Mountain High Stretch
- The Backstroke
- The Breaststroke

MOUNTAIN HIGH STRETCH

Begin here, after doing the Basic Warm-up.

STARTING POSITION: Stand with your feet hip-width apart, your arms hanging by your sides.

STEP 1: Bring both arms forward and up, until they are overhead. Hook your fingers together and turn the palms of your hands up to the ceiling. Pull your shoulders up toward your ears. Inhale as you stretch up.

STEP 2: Keeping your fingers interlaced, press your shoulders down hard. Exhale.

Repeat steps 1 and 2 four times.

STEP 3: Next, still keeping your fingers interlaced, tilt your body to the right. Hold and breathe deeply.

STEP 4: Come upright again and tilt to the left. Hold and breathe deeply.

STEP 5: Come upright again and unhook your fingers. With your wrists flexed, slowly lower your arms out to the sides and return them to the starting position.

Do two complete sets.

POINTER:

◆ Keep your elbows as straight as possible when your fingers are interlocked.

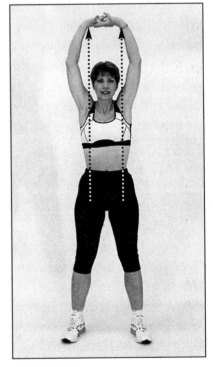

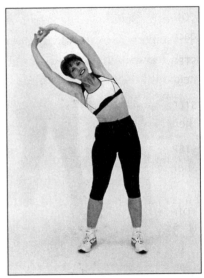

THE BACKSTROKE

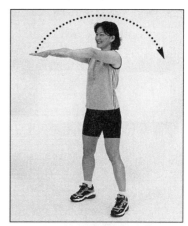

STARTING POSITION: Stand with your feet hip-width apart. Place your arms straight in front of your body at shoulder height.

COUNTS: Every arm circle takes four counts.

STEP 1: Keeping your right arm as straight as possible, circle it back and down, and then return it to the starting position.

STEP 2: As your right arm is on its way down, begin making a similar backward circle with your left arm.

Make four circles with each arm.

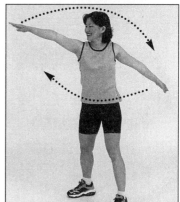

THE BREASTSTROKE

STARTING POSITION: Stand with your feet hip-width apart and your knees slightly bent. Bring your hands together in front of your chest at shoulder height and let your elbows come up and out to the side. Your palms are facing front. Lean forward a tiny bit and look straight ahead.

COUNTS: Every Breaststroke takes four counts, or one count for each movement.

STEP 1: Push your palms forward, keeping them at shoulder height.

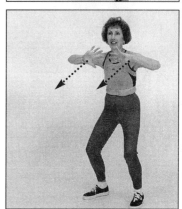

STEP 2: When your arms are fully extended in front of you, circle them out to your sides and simultaneously straighten your legs.

STEP 3: Keeping your legs straight, drop your arms to your sides. Then bend your knees and return to the starting position.

Repeat four times.

POINTERS:

◆ Be sure to spread your arms wide to the side to feel the expanse of the stretch.

◆ This is a great exercise for breathing. Inhale as you move your arms forward and exhale as you return to the starting position.

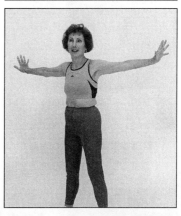

BICYCLING

"Set your own goals and go at your own pace—just keep moving."

—Barbara, seventy-two

When you have survived breast cancer, you can continue to lead the life you love, no matter what age you are. Barbara, an athletic, seventy-two-year-old breast cancer survivor, is proof of this. She bicycles almost every day and also enjoys long walks and downhill skiing. Being active is such a big part of her life that she never would have been happy if she couldn't pursue her favorite outdoor sports. A determined go-getter, she says these activities keep her young and healthy.

Barbara has an excellent gut instinct and pays close attention to her body. When she found an odd dimple in her left breast during a routine self-exam she immediately made appointments to see her internist and gynecologist. Although her condition did not seem alarming, she asked them to be thorough about making a clear diagnosis. So after a mammogram and an ultrasound, she was given a needle biopsy. Since the results were inconclusive, a surgeon performed a tissue biopsy that identified a cancerous growth. Her treatment included a lumpectomy, sentinel lymph node dissection, and radiation therapy.

Barbara's main challenge after her surgery was fatigue. Although she started walking and biking again a few days after surgery, at first she could only move slowly, perspired a lot, and was easily exhausted. Then, after a couple of weeks, she began going faster and farther and felt better. Her surgeon had recommended the Focus on Healing program while Barbara was in the hospital, and within a few weeks she began incorporating it into her recovery. She especially credits the program with helping improve her stamina, which is essential to biking. Today her rides are up to thirty-five miles long.

BIKING SPECIFICS FOR SURVIVORS Bicycling mainly targets the muscles in your legs, buttocks, and hips, so it is not an activity that puts you at great risk for lymphedema or scar tissue tearing. The main stress to the upper body comes from leaning forward on the handlebars for long periods of time.

However, this is easy to remedy. All you need to do is make sure to heed the signals your body is sending you. Occasionally, you should sit up, keep pedaling, and do some Finger Rolls. This is especially important if your hand begins to feel numb or starts to tingle. If these symptoms persist, take a break to give your body a rest, and then continue your ride.

For recreational riders, blood pressure and extreme exhaustion are not likely to be major concerns; competitive riders, however, ought to make a point of monitoring their heart rate (to determine your target heart rate see p. 8). You are probably exercising too hard if your heart is pounding and you are short of breath. Listen to the signals your body sends you about what it needs.

One special note for bikers: If you find that your balance is off when you are riding, stop and walk your bike. You may find it useful to go back and work on the Developing Balance routine in Part Two (p. 101–109).

THE WARM-UP:
- The Basic Warm-up (pp. 15–23)
- Mountain High Stretch
- Overhead Push
- Finger Rolls

MOUNTAIN HIGH STRETCH

Begin here, after doing the Basic Warm-up. Perform this stretch prior to bicycling.

STARTING POSITION: Stand with your feet hip-width apart, your arms hanging by your sides.

STEP 1: Bring both arms forward and up, until they are overhead. Hook your fingers together and turn the palms of your hands up to the ceiling. Pull your shoulders up toward your ears. Inhale as you stretch up.

STEP 2: Keeping your fingers interlaced, press your shoulders down hard. Exhale.

Repeat steps 1 and 2 four times.

STEP 3: Next, still keeping your fingers interlaced, tilt your body to the right. Hold and breathe deeply.

STEP 4: Come upright again and tilt to the left. Hold and breathe deeply.

STEP 5: Come upright again and unhook your fingers. With your wrists flexed, slowly lower your arms out to the sides and return them to the starting position.

Do two complete sets.

POINTER:

◆ Keep your elbows as straight as possible when your fingers are interlocked.

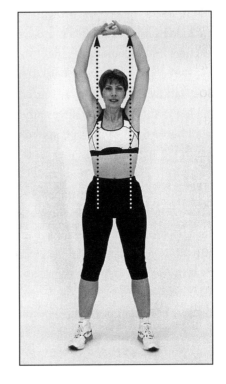

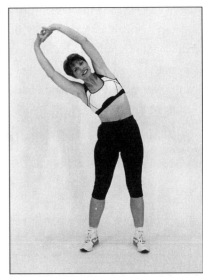

OVERHEAD PUSH

Do this stretch to prepare yourself to put pressure on your hands and wrists and the muscles in your upper body during your ride.

STARTING POSITION: Stand with your feet hip-width apart. Rest your left hand comfortably on your hip. Bend your right elbow so that you bring your right hand up to your right shoulder. Flex your right wrist backward so that your fingers point toward the wall behind you.

COUNTS: Every movement takes four counts.

STEP 1: Bend your knees. As you straighten them, push your right hand up toward the ceiling as if you're a waitress lifting a heavy tray. Keep your arm as close to your head as possible.

STEP 2: Then bend your knees and bring your arm down again. Do not pause at the top.

Repeat four times, then switch arms and do four on the left.

POINTER:

◆ Imagine the sensation of carrying a heavy tray; feeling the resistance makes your muscles work harder and improves the stretch.

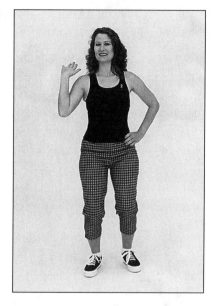

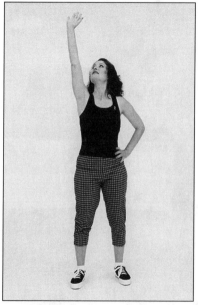

FINGER ROLLS

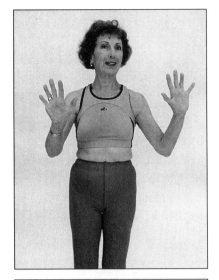

Do Finger Rolls as you bicycle to improve the circulation in your hands, fingers, and arms. It is an antidote for the numbness and tingling you may experience after gripping the handlebars for extended periods of time. You may also stop riding for a few minutes and do this with both hands simultaneously.

STARTING POSITION: Hold on to the handlebars with your left hand. Bring your right hand to your shoulder, palm facing forward with the fingers spread wide.

MOVEMENT: Starting with your little finger, curl your hand into a fist one finger at a time. Rotate the fist to face you. Then open up your fingers one at a time, again starting with your little finger. Then rotate your open palm back to the front.

Repeat with your left hand.

Do four sets of Finger Rolls.

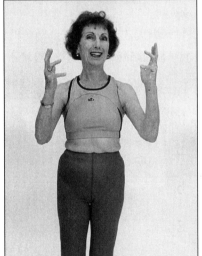

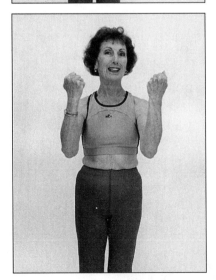

GOLF

$\mathcal{M}$y husband and I had only been married for two years when my cancer was diagnosed. We cried a lot together during my treatment. After my surgery, when I was afraid to look at myself in the mirror, he changed my bandages, emptied my drain, held my hand, and told me I was beautiful. Spending time with my husband is one of my greatest pleasures. In Seattle, where beautiful days are glorious days, we play golf on a course that over-looks mountains and the Pacific Ocean. Though I am not the world's best golfer I do enjoy the sport. I don't like the frustration of missing a shot, but I love walking the fairway and being outdoors.

The hardest part of my physical recovery was the lethargy I felt. When I had completed my radiation therapy I called my brother Marc, who is a surgeon, and asked, "Okay, when do I get my energy back?" He told me it could take up to a year. It was not the news I wanted to hear, but it was reality. So I faithfully did the Focus on Healing program three times a week to increase my range of motion and began a short daily walking routine. Three months later, I went back to the driving range and practiced my swing with a quarter bucket of balls, determined to work my way up to a whole bucket. Soon I was able to play at my own pace, doing exercises between holes because my arm felt stiff. Even today if my arm hurts, gets tired, or feels heavy, I stop playing. I have learned to listen to my body.

As a frequent golfer, I've noticed how different I feel when I take the time to stretch. If I haven't done enough preparation, my arm hurts and throbs after a few holes. Not only does it prevent me from playing, it also produces a certain anxiety. Because I had twenty-three lymph nodes removed, I always worry about the possibility of developing lymphedema. On the other hand, if I spend ten to fifteen minutes patiently stretching in the locker room beforehand, I know I can worry less.

The great thing about Focus on Healing is that it helped me regain my strength and increase my energy. Stretching my scar tissue before I take my first swing with these simple exercises opens up my lymphatic system and chest muscles, and gives me confidence to enjoy the game. I don't have to worry about pulling or tearing something; doing a warm-up puts me in control, not the cancer.

GOLF SPECIFICS FOR SURVIVORS Golf is one of the most challenging sports for breast cancer survivors as it puts stress on the areas in the upper body where surgery has made us vulnerable. Since a golf swing requires a full range of motion and is performed rapidly and with force, we must be certain that we are properly warmed up before we hit the links, paying special attention to prestretching our scar tissue to prevent it from tearing. Before you consider golfing you should be able to successfully complete the entire Ultimate Movements including the Building Strength section.

If you have limited flexibility I don't recommend golfing just yet. But once you have achieved full range of motion, there's generally no reason not to play. However, I do recommend that recent survivors check with their surgeons or radiologists to be sure they are ready.

THE WARM-UP:
- The Basic Warm-up (pp. 15–23)
- Overhead Side Stretch
- Gentle Body Twists
- Shoulder Stretch

OVERHEAD SIDE STRETCH

Begin here, after doing the Basic Warm-up.

WHAT YOU NEED FOR THIS EXERCISE: A golf club.

STARTING POSITION: Stand with your feet hip-width apart. Clasp one end of the golf club in each hand.

STEP 1: Holding the golf club, raise your arms and the club overhead. Gently tilt your body to the right and hold this position for two deep breaths in and out. Return to center.

STEP 2: Now gently tilt your body to the left and hold this position for two deep breaths in and out. Return to center.

Do two sets. Then lower your arms.

POINTERS:

◆ Keep your palms facing outward even at the height of your stretch.

◆ Be gentle and move slowly.

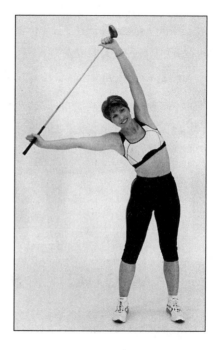

GENTLE BODY TWISTS

Gentle Body Twists wake up the spine and stretch the muscles below your shoulder blades that you will be using for your golf swing.

WHAT YOU NEED FOR THIS EXERCISE: A golf club.

STARTING POSITION: Stand with your feet hip-width apart. Hold your golf club in front of you at shoulder height. Your hands are spread as far apart as possible.

COUNTS: Every twist takes four counts.

STEP 1: Gently turn your upper body to the right.

STEP 2: Rotate back to center and then gently turn to the left. Do four sets.

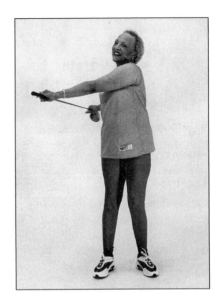

SHOULDER STRETCH

WHAT YOU NEED FOR THIS EXERCISE: A golf club.

STARTING POSITION: Stand with your feet hip-width apart. Grasp the top of the golf club in your right hand.

STEP 1: Lift your right arm and place the golf club behind your back along the spine.

STEP 2: Reach around and grasp the bottom of the golf club in your left hand. Hold the stretch for four deep breaths in and out. Take the opportunity, during the stretch, to bend to your left a little to open up your shoulders. Then release your left hand and bring the club back around. Switch hands and repeat the stretch on the opposite side, bending to the right.

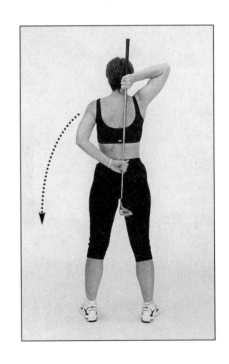

BOWLING

$\mathscr{S}$ally is a forty-two-year-old breast cancer survivor who before she got breast cancer had for years been an avid bowler in a local women's league. She loved the sport and spending time with her teammates, so she eagerly waited to heal from her surgical incision and get through chemotherapy. Finally, eight months after surgery, she went to the lanes and discovered what she most feared. Not only could she not lift a bowling ball with confidence, she couldn't swing her arm back far enough to gain any momentum. It was a terrible outcome and she was heartbroken.

A couple of weeks later Sally attended a presentation I gave near her home and she approached me afterward. More than anything else she wanted to know whether she would ever be able to bowl again. If it was possible, Sally asked, what did she need to do to get there? I persuaded her to join my class.

Together we worked through a plan in stages. It was clear that before Sally would ever be able to pick up her ball she needed to have more strength. And before she could do the exercises to get her strength back, she needed to regain her full range of motion without pain. That meant she had to be able to freely move her arm front, back, up, out, and sideways across her body. After achieving this first goal, she could move on to resistance training with elastic exercise bands to improve her muscle tone and endurance. Based on my experience with other survivors, I told her it would probably take a minimum of six months to reach this goal.

Sally was exceedingly determined and never skipped her exercises in class or at home. By the time six months rolled around she was pain-free, had recovered her complete range of motion, and had built up enough strength to rejoin her league. Almost six months to the day, she went back to bowling. I helped her design the following sport-specific warm-up to do every time she bowled, and she has made a commitment to continue exercising for life so that her scar tissue will stay pliable. It means a lot to Sally to be active, and it makes me happy to know that my program has made such a difference in her life.

BOWLING SPECIFICS FOR SURVIVORS Bowling is an activity that works every part of the body except the neck and head. Swinging the arm low and back is a part of the normal range of motion that most of us don't need to use on a daily basis, and in bowling you add the weight of the ball to this effort. Before you consider bowling you should be able to successfully complete the entire Ultimate Movements including the "Building Strength" section.

Survivors need to be careful about lifting the weight of a bowling ball before they are strong enough. It is important to avoid muscle soreness or micro tears in the muscle tissues. In "Building Strength," go from the least resistant exercise band to the hardest, and make sure you are able to do all of those exercises easily before even attempting to lift a bowling ball. As a bowler you need to be aware of whether you have signs of pain, fatigue, soreness, swelling, and tingling in your hands and arms. When these appear, you should stop and rest and, if they persist, wait until another occasion to bowl.

THE WARM-UP
- The Basic Warm-up (pp. 15–23)
- Around the World
- The Crawl
- The Backstroke
- Overhead Side Stretch
- Chest Expander

AROUND THE WORLD

Begin here, after doing the Basic Warm-up.

STARTING POSITION: Stand with your feet hip-width apart, your arms hanging by your sides.

COUNTS: A complete circle takes four counts.

STEP 1: Bend your knees as you raise your arms forward and overhead.

STEP 2: Straighten your knees as you circle your arms backward and then down to the starting position. Repeat.

STEP 3: Now reverse the circle, bending your knees while bringing your arms back and up behind your head.

STEP 4: Straighten your knees as you circle your arms forward and down to the starting position. Repeat.

POINTER:

◆ The knee bend at the beginning of the movement should feel as if you were about to spring lightly off a diving board.

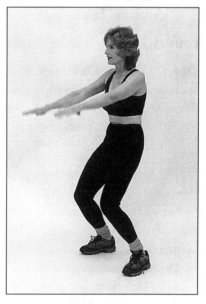

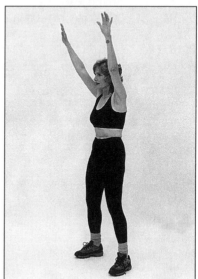

THE CRAWL

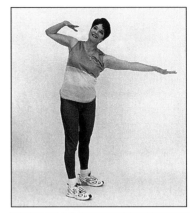

STARTING POSITION: Stand with your feet hip-width apart. Your arms are straight out in front of your body at shoulder height.

COUNTS: Every arm circle takes eight counts.

STEP 1: To do the Crawl, your arms must cycle independently. Lower your right arm down to your side, then bend your right elbow and bring the arm up to shoulder height. From shoulder height, continue the movement by extending the arm straight up in the air.

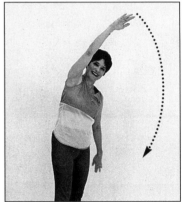

STEP 2: At the same time, bring your left arm down to your side, then bend the left elbow and bring your left arm up to shoulder height. As the left arm is rising, circle the right arm forward and down to the starting position. As the left arm continues straight up into the air, lower your right arm to your side.

Circle both arms four times. Turn your head to the right as your right hand reaches your shoulder and then turn it to the left as your left hand reaches your shoulder. Your movements are continuous and flowing. Try to find a steady rhythm.

POINTER:
◆ Imagine the resistance of the water.

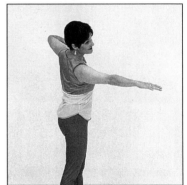

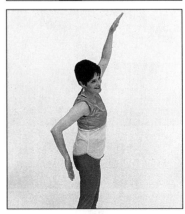

THE BACKSTROKE

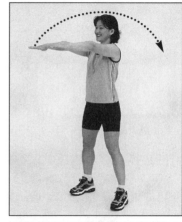

STARTING POSITION: Stand with your feet hip-width apart. Place your arms straight in front of your body at shoulder height.

COUNTS: Each arm circle takes four counts.

STEP 1: Keeping your right arm as straight as possible, circle it back and down, and then return it to the starting position.

STEP 2: As your right arm is on its way down, begin making a similar backward circle with your left arm.

Make four circles with each arm.

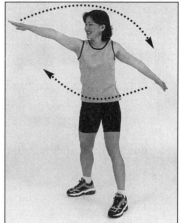

OVERHEAD
SIDE STRETCH

STARTING POSITION: Stand with your feet hip-width apart, your arms hanging by your sides with the palms facing inward.

STEP 1: Swing your right arm slowly out to the side and up over your head. Your palm should be facing out. Gently tilt your body to the left and reach to the left with your right arm. Hold this position for two deep breaths in and out.

STEP 2: Return your body to an upright position and bring your right arm back down, making a slow, reaching arc.

Repeat the stretch on your left side.

Do two more stretches on each side.

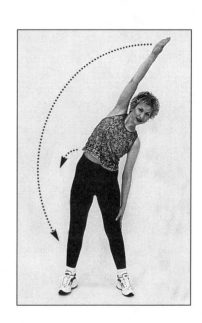

POINTERS:

◆ Keep your palm facing outward even at the height of the stretch.

◆ Be gentle and move slowly.

CHEST EXPANDER

WHAT YOU NEED FOR THIS EXERCISE: An elastic exercise band without handles.

STARTING POSITION: Place the elastic band around your back where your bra strap goes, as if you are measuring your bust line with a measuring tape. Hold the band in an overhanded grip with your hands directly in front of your armpits. Make sure the band is on the outside of your arms. The ends should dangle from your thumbs not your little fingers.

COUNTS: Every movement takes two counts.

STEP 1: Push your hands directly forward until your elbows are straight.

STEP 2: Then let the band pull your straight arms out to the sides and back, expanding your chest. Breathe in deeply.

STEP 3: Reverse directions by pulling your straight arms back to the front. Then bring your hands back to your armpits.
 Repeat. Build up to four repetitions, as you get stronger.

POINTERS:

◆ You will probably need to experiment with how much slack you need on your band in order to reach the full extension forward.

◆ Do not allow the band to touch any part of your arms when they are open to the sides.

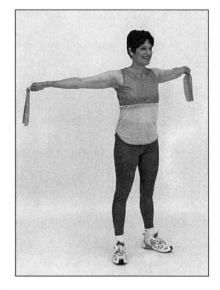

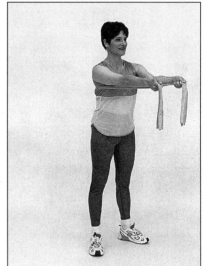

AEROBICS

"Never give up. Don't stop living and doing the things you love, just pay more attention to your body, maybe do them slower, but never give up."

—*Terri, forty-five*

Terri has an indomitable spirit and she's thriving. Everywhere she goes she spreads laughter and a positive attitude. Still, it took sheer determination to overcome the trauma of cancer and cancer treatment. She began doing Focus on Healing as a four-year survivor to maintain her range of motion and warm up for her other activities. When she joined the program I learned that she had undergone three surgeries and chemotherapy, and despite severe exhaustion remained active throughout. After surgery, a personal trainer with specialized knowledge of breast cancer and lymphedema had introduced

Terri to aerobics, keeping in mind her physical limitations. At age forty-five, she credits those aerobics classes with filling her with an energy she hasn't felt since childhood.

During chemotherapy, Terri trained with light weights and walked. Some days it was hard to put one foot in front of the other because the chemicals wore her out. From the beginning she went to a physical therapist twice a week and practiced her stretches religiously. Reconstruction a year later threw off her balance and she also lost mobility in her arm. When she started doing aerobics, it took her weeks to last even ten minutes. Nevertheless, she was motivated to persist. She made a point to keep her arm low and concentrate on her legs. Ultimately she could finish a whole class. Even now she always stops and rests when she feels tired or sore. She attributes her success in part to knowing her true limits.

It took another year for Terri to feel comfortable mentally as well as physically. She always knew that she would never be the same on the outside—and even on the inside—but also that she would get better and in time be okay. She wasn't going to let anything stop her from doing what she loved. As a result of her cancer experience, she feels that she has more to offer other people now than ever before. Today she is a certified Focus on Healing instructor teaching at a hospital in Everett, Washington.

AEROBICS SPECIFICS FOR SURVIVORS Aerobics provide an excellent cardiovascular workout that works all your muscles, including those of your arms, shoulders, and chest. However, it includes a few potential problems. If you are at risk for lymphedema, please be aware that this activity may trigger swelling. When your blood pressure goes up during class, a compromised lymphatic system has to work harder. Aerobics movements are often repetitive and this likewise creates stress. You should also bear in mind that low-impact aerobics are safer than high-impact aerobics.

Before you consider doing aerobics you should be able to successfully complete the entire Ultimate Movements workout including the "Building Strength" section. Pay attention to the signals of your body. Lower your arms if they feel heavy or ache. Many survivors develop numbness around their surgical sites. When you have no sensation, you can hurt yourself without realizing it. So please exercise with caution and consult your physician, physical therapist, or occupational therapist before pursuing an aerobics program.

THE WARM-UP
◆ The Basic Warm-up (pp. 15–23)
◆ Mountain High Stretch
◆ The Crawl
◆ The Backstroke
◆ The Breaststroke
◆ Overhead Side Stretch

MOUNTAIN HIGH STRETCH

Begin here, after doing the Basic Warm-up.

STARTING POSITION: Stand with your feet hip-width apart, your arms hanging by your sides.

STEP 1: Bring both arms forward and up, until they are overhead. Hook your fingers together and turn the palms of your hands up to the ceiling. Pull your shoulders up toward your ears. Inhale as you stretch up.

STEP 2: Keeping your fingers interlaced, press your shoulders down hard. Exhale.

Repeat steps 1 and 2 four times.

STEP 3: Next, still keeping your fingers interlaced, tilt your body to the right. Hold and breathe deeply.

STEP 4: Come upright again and tilt to the left. Hold and breathe deeply.

STEP 5: Come upright again and unhook your fingers. With your wrists flexed, slowly lower your arms out to the sides and return them to the starting position.

Do two complete sets.

POINTER:
◆ Keep your elbows as straight as possible when your fingers are interlocked.

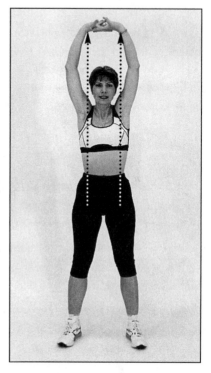

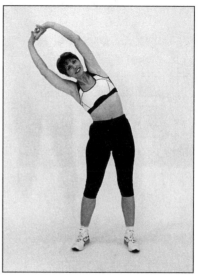

THE CRAWL

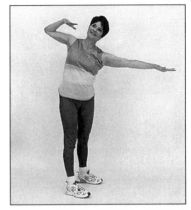

STARTING POSITION: Stand with your feet hip-width apart. Your arms are straight out in front of your body at shoulder height.

COUNTS: Every arm circle takes eight counts.

STEP 1: To do the Crawl, your arms must cycle independently. Lower your right arm down to your side, then bend your right elbow and bring the arm up to shoulder height. From shoulder height, continue the movement by extending the arm straight up in the air.

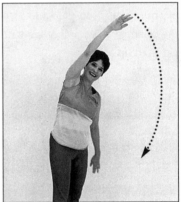

STEP 2: At the same time, bring your left arm down to your side, then bend the left elbow and bring your left arm up to shoulder height. As the left arm is rising, circle the right arm forward and down to the starting position. As the left arm continues straight up into the air, lower your right arm to your side.

Circle both arms four times. Turn your head to the right as your right hand reaches your shoulder and then turn it to the left as your left hand reaches your shoulder. Your movements are continuous and flowing. Try to find a steady rhythm.

POINTER:

◆ Imagine the resistance of the water.

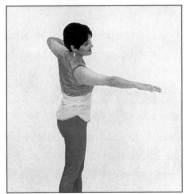

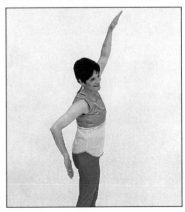

THE BACKSTROKE

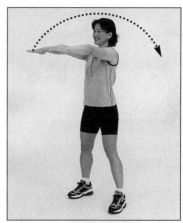

STARTING POSITION: Stand with your feet hip-width apart. Place your arms straight in front of your body at shoulder height.

COUNTS: Every arm circle takes four counts.

STEP 1: Keeping your right arm as straight as possible, circle it back and down, and then return it to the starting position.

STEP 2: As your right arm is on its way down, begin making a similar backward circle with your left arm.

Make four circles with each arm.

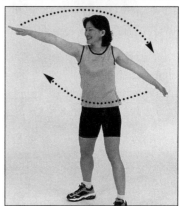

THE BREASTSTROKE

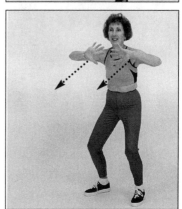

STARTING POSITION: Stand with your feet hip-width apart and your knees slightly bent. Bring your hands together in front of your chest at shoulder height and let your elbows come up and out to the side. Your palms are facing front. Lean forward a tiny bit and look straight ahead.

COUNTS: Every Breaststroke takes four counts, or one count for each movement.

STEP 1: Push your palms forward, keeping them at shoulder height.

STEP 2: When your arms are fully extended in front of you, circle them out to your sides and simultaneously straighten your legs.

STEP 3: Keeping your legs straight, drop your arms to your sides. Then bend your knees and return to the starting position.

Repeat four times.

POINTERS:

◆ Be sure to spread your arms wide to the side to feel the expanse of the stretch.

◆ This is a great exercise for breathing. Inhale as you move your arms forward and exhale as you return to the starting position.

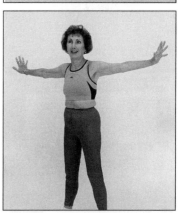

OVERHEAD SIDE STRETCH

STARTING POSITION: Stand with your feet hip-width apart; your arms hanging by your sides with the palms facing inward.

STEP 1: Swing your right arm slowly out to the side and up over your head. Your palm should be facing out. Gently tilt your body to the left and reach to the left with your right arm. Hold this position for two deep breaths in and out.

STEP 2: Return your body to an upright position and bring your right arm back down, making a slow, reaching arc.

Repeat the stretch on your left side.

Do two more stretches on each side.

POINTERS:

◆ Keep your palm facing outward even at the height of the stretch.

◆ Be gentle and move slowly.

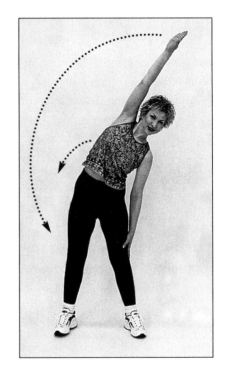

WEIGHT TRAINING

*J*anet is a forty-seven-year-old survivor of breast cancer who trains with weights three times a week and participates in dragon boating, a competitive team rowing sport created in Canada specifically for breast cancer survivors. Her surgery in the fall of 1998 went well, after which she underwent twenty-five radiation treatments. As a nurse, she understood the importance of exercise to her recovery process and sought out special assistance at a wellness center near her home. Being active during the period of her radiation therapy helped her focus on the future and push through the discomfort, although the sessions themselves were tough.

The thing Janet wanted most right then was to get on with her life. She wanted to be able to put cancer behind her and avoid having to think about it anymore. The hardest aspect of recovery though was suddenly finding her treatment done and feeling alone. No longer was she receiving constant medical attention and direction, and she felt a little lost.

At the wellness center she worked with a physical therapist experienced in the unique needs of breast cancer survivors. Her trainer designed a special program for Janet using free weights, weight machines, and cardio machines that helped her build back her strength and gave her an emotional lift. Some days she didn't want to go to the center because she felt drained, but when she got there she was always glad she did. She could be around other people while she worked out and found the weight training gave her emotional balance as well as physical improvements. In time she took up guitar lessons and singing. She grew from her cancer experience and learned to look at life through different eyes.

Janet took care of her emotional needs in part by connecting with other breast cancer survivors in Focus on Healing classes, on retreats, and by joining a dragon boating team. At the hospital where she works she has since become the liaison to other women going through cancer surgery and treatment. As the contact for the Reach to Recovery program, she feels as if she is giving back to all those who helped her make it through.

WEIGHT TRAINING SPECIFICS FOR SURVIVORS

Weight training can target and train all of your muscles, including those of the shoulders, arms, chest, sides, and back. However, if you're going to use weights you ought to get the advice of an informed physical therapist. A trainer who has experience working with women with surgical scar tissue who have had node dissection can help you maximize your training without causing or exacerbating lymphedema or any other injury. You may have to search for an appropriate trainer, but it's well worth it. Ask at your gym or seek a referral from other survivors (also see Resources).

Please be aware that in general the National Lymphedema Network doesn't recommend using a weight of more than fifteen pounds because of the pulling stress on the muscles. You should start with much lower weights than that, particularly if you are not in good physical shape. If you lift too heavy a weight before you are ready you can get muscle soreness or micro tears in your muscle tissues. Both of these would activate the lymphatic system to assist in muscle repair or the removal of cellular waste (lactic acid). The repetitiveness of weighted exercises may also be problematic for some survivors because it pumps up your circulatory system. Before you consider weight training you should be able to successfully complete the entire Ultimate Movements workout including the "Building Strength" section.

THE WARM-UP:

◆ The Basic Warm-up (pp. 15–23)
◆ Mountain High Stretch
◆ Overhead Side Stretch
◆ The Backstroke
◆ The Breaststroke
◆ Chest and Shoulder Stretch

MOUNTAIN HIGH STRETCH

Begin here, after doing the Basic Warm-up.

STARTING POSITION: Stand with your feet hip-width apart, your arms hanging by your sides.

STEP 1: Bring both arms forward and up, until they are overhead. Hook your fingers together and turn the palms of your hands up to the ceiling. Pull your shoulders up toward your ears. Inhale as you stretch up.

STEP 2: Keeping your fingers interlaced, press your shoulders down hard. Exhale.

Repeat steps 1 and 2 four times.

STEP 3: Next, still keeping your fingers interlaced, tilt your body to the right. Hold and breathe deeply.

STEP 4: Come upright again and tilt to the left. Hold and breathe deeply.

STEP 5: Come upright again and unhook your fingers. With your wrists flexed, slowly lower your arms out to the sides and return them to the starting position.

Do two complete sets.

POINTER:
◆ Keep your elbows as straight as possible when your fingers are interlocked.

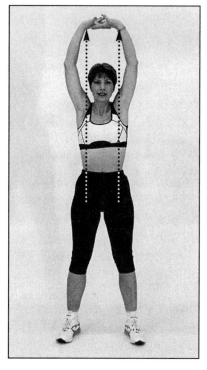

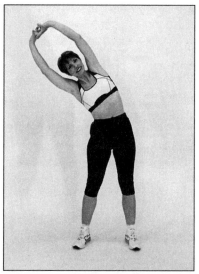

OVERHEAD SIDE STRETCH

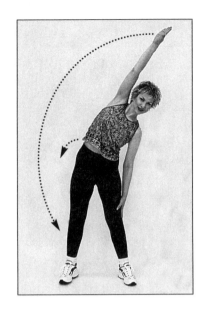

STARTING POSITION: Stand with your feet hip-width apart, your arms hanging by your sides with the palms facing inward.

STEP 1: Swing your right arm slowly out to the side and up over your head. Your palm should be facing out. Gently tilt your body to the left and reach to the left with your right arm. Hold this position for two deep breaths in and out.

STEP 2: Return your body to an upright position and bring your right arm back down, making a slow, reaching arc.

Repeat the stretch on your left side.

Do two more stretches on each side.

POINTERS:

◆ Keep your palm facing outward even at the height of the stretch.

◆ Be gentle and move slowly.

THE BACKSTROKE

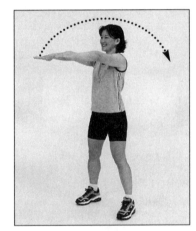

STARTING POSITION: Stand with your feet hip-width apart. Place your arms straight in front of your body at shoulder height.

COUNTS: Every arm circle takes four counts.

STEP 1: Keeping your right arm as straight as possible, circle it back and down, and then return it to the starting position.

STEP 2: As your right arm is on its way down, begin making a similar backward circle with your left arm.

Make four circles with each arm.

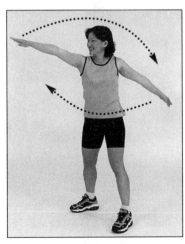

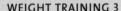

THE BREASTSTROKE

STARTING POSITION: Stand with your feet hip-width apart and your knees slightly bent. Bring your hands together in front of your chest at shoulder height and let your elbows come up and out to the side. Your palms are facing front. Lean forward a tiny bit and look straight ahead.

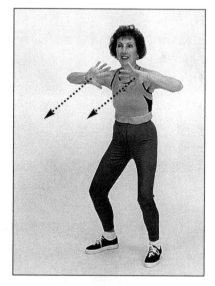

COUNTS: Every Breaststroke takes four counts, or one count for each movement.

STEP 1: Push your palms forward, keeping them at shoulder height.

STEP 2: When your arms are fully extended in front of you, circle them out to your sides and simultaneously straighten your legs.

STEP 3: Keeping your legs straight, drop your arms to your sides. Then bend your knees and return to the starting position.
   Repeat four times.

POINTERS:

◆ Be sure to spread your arms wide to the side to feel the expanse of the stretch.

◆ This is a great exercise for breathing. Inhale as you move your arms forward and exhale as you return to the starting position.

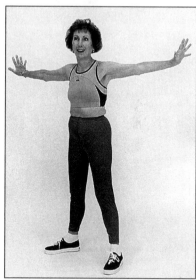

CHEST AND SHOULDER STRETCH

STARTING POSITION: Stand with your feet hip-width apart. Interlace your fingers behind your lower back with your palms facing up.

STEP 1: Straighten your arms as much as you can and inhale deeply while lifting your chest up and forward. Press your shoulders all the way back and down. Exaggerate the position by thinking about your shoulder blades coming together. Hold the position for two more deep breaths in and out.

STEP 2: Keeping your hands clasped, relax the position and slump your shoulders forward. Exhale.

Repeat the stretch four times.

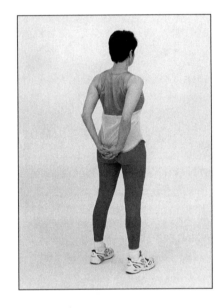

TENNIS

"Because we need to stay healthy to fight illness, it is very important that we survivors keep fit. I want to be around to see my kids grow up!"
—*Dana, forty-eight*

*D*ana found a small lump in her right breast soon after she stopped nursing her infant son. She watched it for a couple of months and then went for a mammogram. Her doctor gave her the option of doing a needle biopsy and was clearly surprised at the results. "I can't believe it, but there are cancer cells." She was thirty-six years old. The diagnosis arrived on her baby's first birthday.

Dana was willing to do whatever it took to survive and be around for her two young children and her husband. She had a mastectomy and node dissection followed by six chemotherapy treatments. For the next two years she did not do any organized sporting activities. Her children were one and three years old and they kept her incredibly busy. Then she and her husband began biking together and she took up jogging on her own. Back in high school Dana had played tennis and liked it. Now she sought out a friend to be her regular tennis partner. That was ten years ago. This year she joined a U.S. Tennis Association team in Seattle.

Dana is currently working on losing the fifty pounds she gained since getting married, having two babies, and coping with her fatigue and treatment. At the same time, she is actually fitter and more in control of her body. Dana loves exercise—especially tennis. The sport offers her a good way to socialize and it never bores her; playing with her team contributes to her health and happiness.

TENNIS SPECIFICS FOR SURVIVORS Tennis is a very rapid and vigorous sport in which you run around a lot, thus it poses potential concerns similar to those of an aerobics program (see Aerobics Specifics for Survivors, p. 218). In addition, although every muscle group, from head to toe, is getting a solid workout as you run around the courts, the game puts specific stresses on your arms, chest, and shoulders—hence the injury "tennis elbow." As a survivor, you need to take your unique circumstances into account in order to participate safely. Before you consider playing tennis you should be able to successfully complete the entire Ultimate Movements workout, including the "Building Strength" section.

Tennis is not recommended for survivors who are still in treatment or have only recently been in treatment. It is important to give your scar tissue a chance to heal properly and then make sure you have full range of motion before picking up a racquet again. Once you are fully healed, you can begin with gentle volleying over the net and then work your way back to more competitive matches. The Focus on Healing program can help you rebuild your strength and stamina. As with any form of exercise you undertake, take it easy when you feel tired, sore, or have tingling in your hands and arms.

If you have lymphedema, you should compression wrap your arm while playing. You must learn to judge what is going to provoke a flare-up and then manage the consequences. Decide for yourself how often you can play, when you should be less aggressive, and how much recovery time to allow between days on the court. It can be difficult to pull back when playing a competitive sport, but your health is worth it.

THE WARM-UP
- The Basic Warm-up (pp. 15–23)
- Overhead Side Stretch
- Shoulder Stretch
- The Crawl
- The Backstroke

OVERHEAD SIDE STRETCH

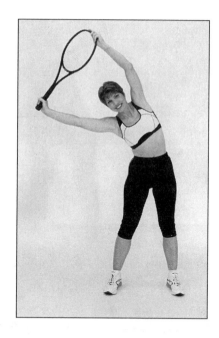

Begin here, after doing the Basic Warm-up.

WHAT YOU NEED FOR THIS EXERCISE: A tennis racquet.

STARTING POSITION: Stand with your feet hip-width apart. Grip the top and bottom of your tennis racquet with your hands.

STEP 1: Holding the ends of the racquet, raise your arms overhead. Gently tilt your body to the right and hold this position for two deep breaths in and out. Return to center.

STEP 2: Now gently tilt your body to the left and hold this position for two deep breaths in and out. Return to center.
    Do two sets. Then lower your arms.

POINTER:

 Be gentle and move slowly.

SHOULDER STRETCH

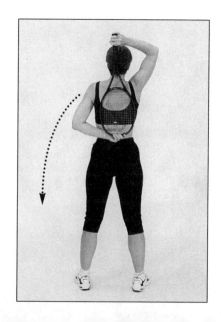

WHAT YOU NEED FOR THIS EXERCISE: A tennis racquet.

STARTING POSITION: Stand with your feet hip-width apart. Grasp the top of the tennis racquet in your right hand.

STEP 1: Lift your right arm and lower the tennis racquet behind your back along the spine.

STEP 2: Reach your left arm behind you and grasp the bottom of the tennis racquet in your left hand. Hold the stretch for four deep breaths in and out. Take the opportunity, during the stretch, to bend to your left a little to open up your shoulders. Then release your left hand and lower the racquet.

STEP 3: Switch hands and repeat the stretch on the opposite side, bending to the right.

231

THE CRAWL

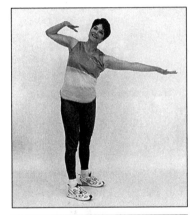

STARTING POSITION: Stand with your feet hip-width apart. Your arms should be straight out in front of your body at shoulder height.

COUNTS: Every arm circle takes eight counts.

STEP 1: To do the Crawl, your arms must cycle independently. Lower your right arm down to your side, then bend your right elbow and bring the arm up to shoulder height. From shoulder height, continue the movement by extending the arm straight up in the air.

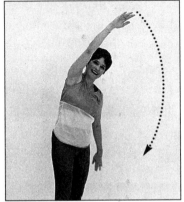

STEP 2: At the same time, bring your left arm down to your side, then bend the left elbow and bring your left arm up to shoulder height. As the left arm is rising, circle the right arm forward and down to the starting position. As the left arm continues straight up into the air, lower your right arm to your side.

Circle both arms four times. Turn your head to the right as your right hand reaches your shoulder and then turn it to the left as your left hand reaches your shoulder. Your movements are continuous and flowing. Try to find a steady rhythm.

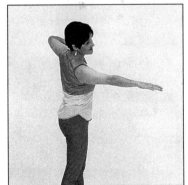

POINTER:
◆ Imagine the resistance of the water.

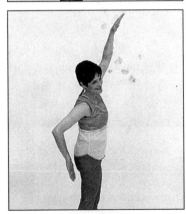

THE BACKSTROKE

STARTING POSITION: Stand with your feet hip-width apart. Place your arms straight in front of your body at shoulder height.

COUNTS: Every arm circle takes four counts.

STEP 1: Keeping your right arm as straight as possible, circle it back and down, and then return it to the starting position.

STEP 2: As your right arm is on its way down, begin making a similar backward circle with your left arm.

Make four circles with each arm.

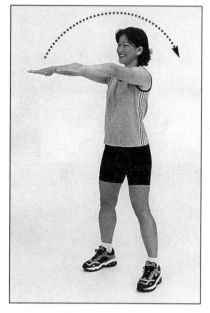

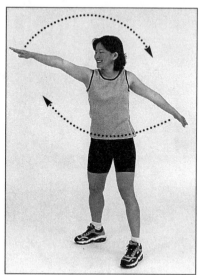

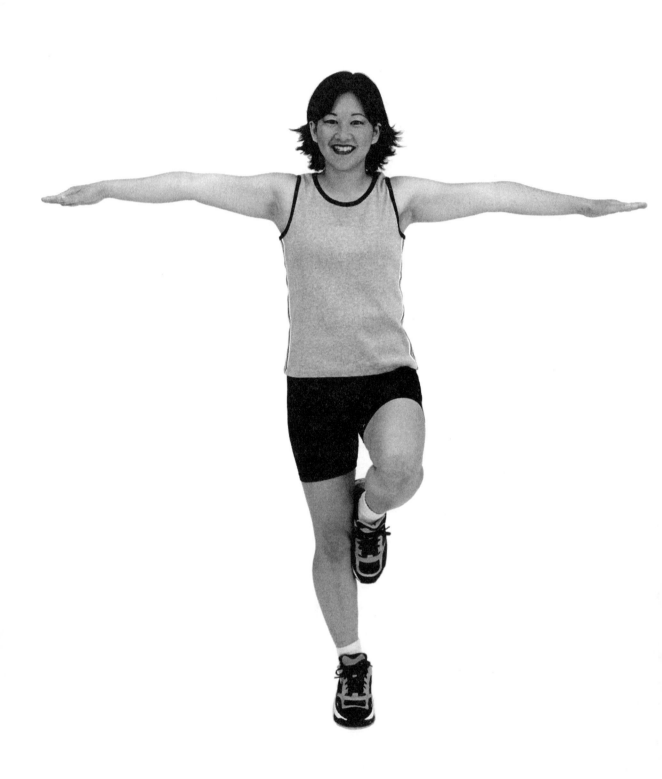

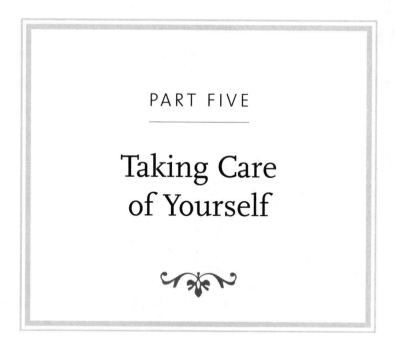

PART FIVE

Taking Care
of Yourself

Recovering from breast cancer is a journey that begins the moment you are diagnosed and continues for the rest of your life. It is not easy. It is also not something that any of us would have chosen to experience. But I know you can thrive after cancer. In fact, the experience may even fade into the background of your life. Until that day, it is important to do everything you can to support your healing process. You deserve it!

By now, you have already begun practicing an exercise routine from Part Two, "Adjusting to the Needs of Your New Body," or Part Three, "The Ultimate Movements." Exercise is one of the best tools of recovery because it helps you cope with both the physical and emotional issues that follow surgery and come up during chemotherapy and radiation therapy. But exercise is not the only tool that is available to you.

So in the next six chapters, I am going to discuss some of the other ways you can nurture yourself and find the help you need to feel better. Consider this information an adjunct to the Focus on Healing program, and remember that your needs today may be different from tomorrow.

Because these are the subjects that are most often discussed by the women in my classes, the chapters in Part Five, "Taking Care of Yourself," include:

◆ Nutrition and Weight Control
◆ Prosthetic Breasts
◆ Coping with Radiation Therapy
◆ Coping with Chemotherapy
◆ Mammography and Self-examination After Breast Cancer Diagnosis
◆ Finding Support

NUTRITION AND WEIGHT CONTROL

*T*here used to be an old joke that the one good thing about cancer is that it helps you lose weight. However, weight gain is now one of the many side effects of cancer treatment. Weight gain is particularly common in breast cancer patients. Although chemotherapy can make you feel nauseated, there are many antinausea drugs available today, so loss of appetite is frequently not as big an issue as it once was. The steroids in chemotherapy "cocktails" can also induce weight gain. Furthermore, some of the drug therapies now prescribed by doctors to inhibit the spread of cancer after surgery may induce modest weight gain. Studies show that this weight gain is not significant. This all makes it harder to maintain your ideal weight.

Other factors that typically contribute to weight gain are stress and fatigue. Many people eat as a reaction to the emotional stress of diagnosis and treatment. Fatigue during and for many months after treatment is very common. Naturally you may sleep more and move less during this period. Even if you eat the same amount of food that you did pretreatment, you can put on weight, as inactivity results in fewer calories being burned.

I have struggled with my weight ever since my cancer treatment, even though I get plenty of exercise each week and teach Focus on Healing. To cope, I must be careful about what I eat. Once you gain weight, it can be hard to lose unless you make a conscious effort to do so. For weight control, I recommend doing the Basic Warm-up and the Ultimate Movements three times a week. Until you are ready for the Ultimate Movements, substitute one of the fitness programs in Part Two, "Adjusting to the Needs of Your New Body." Exercise is one of the best metabolism boosters available.

So what should survivors eat during and after treatment? And in addition to exercise, how else can we cope with our weight gain? I investigated these and other questions with Suzanne Dixon, an epidemiologist and dietitian at the University of Michigan Comprehensive Cancer Center. The following are a few general guidelines.

NUTRITION DURING TREATMENT Doctors recommend that cancer survivors make every attempt to maintain their original weight during radiation and chemotherapy. Dieting is inappropriate at this time because you need full caloric and nutritional intake to recover from surgery and fight your illness. There are, however, ways to alter your diet to boost your metabolism and reduce your intake of unhealthy fats. A nutritionist or dietitian can help you manage your weight appropriately and help you tailor your diet for this purpose. For advice on finding a professional, refer to the resources section.

When weight comes off during treatment, it most likely means that you are losing muscle mass. Loss of muscle can make it harder to function and decrease your energy. But since muscles burn more calories per pound than fat, it also sets you up for weight gain later on. Exercise helps you maintain muscle mass so you should do your best to remain active. When you feel able, you can practice the routines in this book.

If you feel nauseated, try keeping some food in your stomach at all times. Nibble throughout the day, but keep the portions modest. Eating frequent small meals has the added benefit of boosting your metabolism so you actually burn more calories. Rather than allowing your metabolic "engine" to shut down during the lengthy stretches between meals, you keep it charged and running by giving it a little bit to work on throughout the day. Should you feel fatigued, make sure to include some protein or fat in every meal. Protein and fats provide longer-lasting energy than carbohydrates. Good sources are eggs, chicken, fish, cottage cheese, and yogurt. Try eating a piece of whole grain bread with peanut butter on it.

Your medicine may give you constipation. Prunes, prune juice, and raisins can help loosen your stools, as well as foods that contain insoluble fiber. Sources of insoluble fiber include wheat bran cereals, the skin of apples, the stringy part of celery, and other tough parts of plants. If you have the opposite problem—diarrhea—soluble fiber is the antidote. Soluble fiber is sticky, gooey fiber. Examples include oatmeal, white rice, mashed potatoes, and bananas.

More and more research is showing the importance of having a healthy population of friendly bacteria in your intestinal tract. Life-enhancing bacteria, such as *lactobacillus acidophilus,* are called probiotics and they keep your digestive system running smoothly. Yogurt is one good source, as are miso soup, sauerkraut, and other fermented products. You can also find probiotic supplements in most health food stores and vitamin shops.

Perhaps most important, always drink plenty of fresh water. This helps you flush chemicals out of your body, keeps you energized, and contributes to weight maintenance.

GENERAL NUTRITION Although in controlled studies, diet has not been shown to promote healing, good nutrition is an important factor in everyone's overall health. Plant-based diets that contain plenty of fresh fruits and vegetables are the best because they contain numerous important nutrients called phytochemicals (*phyto* means "plant"). While everyone would benefit from eating more fruits and vegetables to get adequate amounts of phytochemicals, the minimum number of servings of fruits and vegetables you should eat every day is five. This may sound like a lot, but remember, a serving is only half a cup of most vegetables, one cup (loosely packed) of green leafy vegetables, one-quarter to half a cup

of berries, or an ounce of dried fruit. If you focus on including these foods in meals and snacks, you can easily reach this goal.

Changing everything you eat would be an overwhelming chore. What works better is to focus on what is missing from your diet rather than what's in your diet. Do not focus on cutting foods out. Instead, focus on all the healthy things you need to add in. So instead of running out and becoming a vegetarian—unless you already are one—simply add fruits and vegetables, and whole grains and legumes into your meals and snacks more often. Not only will you get valuable phytonutrients in this manner, it can also help you keep your weight under control. Picture a large fast-food hamburger. It contains about 700 calories. To get the same number of calories from fruits, vegetables, and beans, you would have to eat plates of them. They are a healthy and less fattening alternative, because they have fewer calories for the given volume of food.

There is no specific food that is off limits as far as cancer and health goes. Rather, the research demonstrates that lack of healthy plant foods—fruits, vegetables, whole grains, and legumes—is a much bigger problem than the presence of specific "bad" foods. You should eat a well-balanced diet of healthy foods that give you enough protein, carbohydrates, vitamins, and minerals. By healthy foods I mean those that are not pumped full of sugar, preservatives, and other chemicals. Some particular foods that are not so great include saturated fats, red or fatty meat, cheese, whole milk, ice cream, fast foods, snack foods, and microwavable foods. That's why, for snacks and meals, I recommend incorporating nuts, seeds, legumes, whole grains, olive oil, canola oil, fish, and flaxseed into your diet instead of those other ingredients.

GETTING HELP There are no easy answers to weight control. But focusing on eating healthy and leading an active lifestyle definitely helps. Here are a few ideas:

◆ Talk to your doctor about your issues with your weight.
◆ Seek out a professional nutritionist or dietitian (see Resources).
◆ Join a weight-loss group.
◆ Read *The Cancer Survival Cookbook* or *What to Eat Now* (see Recommended Reading).

TIPS FOR WEIGHT CONTROL In addition to eating more plant foods, Suzanne Dixon suggests the following tips for weight management:

FILL UP ON FIBER. Fiber does three things for weight control. First, it helps fill you up faster, so you eat fewer calories. Second, it slows down the pace at which your body converts food into fuel. Thus you feel full longer and eat less over the course of the day. Third, new research suggests that people who consume a lot of fiber actually absorb fewer calories from the foods they eat.

WATER, WATER EVERYWHERE. Drink water before each snack and meal. Drink water throughout the day. Water fills you up and therefore you want to eat less. We also sometimes mistake the signals the body sends us about being thirsty for being hungry. So if you keep your body well-hydrated by drinking a lot of water, you can get rid of the "I'm thirsty" signals. Then, when your body tells you to eat, you know that it's really food that your body wants.

Before each meal and snack, before you put any food into your mouth, stop and first drink eight to sixteen ounces of plain water. Wait fifteen minutes. Then eat. Waiting allows your brain to register that your body has received the water.

SET BEHAVIOR-BASED GOALS. People who use behavior-based goals for motivation, rather than goals such as numbers on a scale, have more success with weight loss and weight control. Do not say "I'm going to lose twenty pounds," for example, or "I'm going to fit into that outfit in one month." Instead, set goals, such as "I will exercise three times this week," "I will eat three servings of fruit and three servings of vegetables today," or "I will bring fruit to snack on at work this week."

This way, any time you don't reach your goal, you can figure out why and come up with new strategies for fixing the problem. Maybe you didn't exercise because you were too tired after work. One possible solution is to do your exercise first thing in the morning. Another way to fit in exercise would be to take a walk at lunch.

THINK POSITIVE: Frame your diet goals in positive terms. Do not say "I can't have any chocolate," for example, or "I will never eat hamburgers again." This just focuses your attention on what you cannot have. Instead, say "I can add in two servings of vegetables today to improve my diet and help myself lose weight."

LOVE YOURSELF. Research shows that the more you dislike your body, the less likely you are to succeed at losing weight and keeping it off. It is not self-supporting to say "I'm so fat, I'll never reach my goal weight," or "I'm too heavy to exercise. I'll just look silly." Instead, begin to accept yourself as you are. Look at all the wonderful things that your body can do for you now. Then design a diet-and-exercise program that you can stick to.

PROSTHETIC BREASTS

*T*he benefits of prosthetic breasts—breast forms—are several. First are the aesthetic benefits. They substitute for the appearance of missing breasts by filling out our clothes, thereby helping us feel feminine and attractive. A well-fitted breast form can go a long way toward renewing self-esteem after the loss of an original breast.

In addition, breast forms have therapeutic benefits. They help us maintain our spinal alignment and center of balance. Many of us experience difficulty with our posture after surgery. Our muscles have naturally become accustomed to carrying a specific and equal distribution of weight. Therefore, when we undergo a shift in that distribution, we often begin tilting or dropping our shoulders. This can lead to neck and back pain and a whole host of related ailments. Furthermore, we can lose our sense of grace and become clumsy. Well-designed prosthetic breasts match the weight of our missing breasts as closely as possible, thereby protecting us from pain and accidents.

Let me pause here and state unequivocally that a woman's breasts do not define her beauty. Our culture places far too much emphasis on appearance and celebrates certain features over others. Nonetheless, your breasts are part of your sexual identity, as they have been since puberty—not to mention a part of your body. You may have a host of reactions to the loss of a breast. No two women will have an identical response. You are entitled to each and every one of your feelings. You are also entitled to do whatever makes you feel whole and feminine, including wearing a breast form.

Of course, you may have personal issues with prosthetic breasts. Some women find them embarrassing. They find exercising in health clubs with their prostheses both physically and socially awkward. They don't want other women to look at them changing in the dressing room. They also worry about their breast forms shifting during movement. It is an individual decision whether or not to wear a breast form. By choosing not to wear one, however, it means that you may need to work harder to stretch and strengthen your muscles. This is the main reason I advocate wearing them.

Personally, I choose to look at prosthetic breasts as both helpful and occasionally humorous. One survivor I know went swimming and then left her breast form hanging on the fan in her guest bedroom to dry. Because she started wearing her spare one, she forgot about it. At the conclusion of a long visit, her father summoned up his courage and told her, "I don't know how to say this, but I think you should know that there's a breast in my room." Can you imagine how this man felt staring at it for ten nights?

Another woman I know came home from work one hot and humid evening and tore off her breast form because she felt so sweaty and tired. Usually she would put it in a box, but this evening she just tossed it on the sofa. Her dog immediately jumped up, snatched her breast, and started running around the house using it as a chew toy. When her husband heard her screaming and chasing the dog, he came flying up the stairs in alarm. Needless to say, she's now more careful where she leaves her breast form.

PAYING FOR A PROSTHESIS Good news: Many insurance companies will pay for your prosthesis and your specialized bra with a written prescription from a doctor. Retailers are familiar with these benefits, so remember to ask about them when you schedule an appointment to be fitted. Women without insurance have options, too: contacting the patient services department at their local chapter of the American Cancer Society for assistance in securing their prostheses free of charge or for a nominal fee (see Resources).

GETTING FITTED After surgery, you may feel uncomfortable wearing a bra until your incision has healed and your swelling has subsided. In the meantime there are a couple of postoperative undergarments to choose from. The first is a *softee*, a snug cotton camisole without inseams. The second is a *leisure bra*, which has hooks in front for easy access and longer elastic around the bust line. Your physician can tell you when it is appropriate to go for a fitting for a more permanent bra and breast form.

The next step is finding a good fitter. Not everyone has the right training or sensibility. Some stores, however—Nordstrom is one—give employees special training and certification (see Resources). You can also call around to local retailers before you visit to see if they have a similar program and/or specially trained staff. Or your local American Cancer Society chapter should be able to guide you to a good fitter. It is important to know where to go to have a positive experience before you shop. My own story is a perfect example of why.

Following my lumpectomy, I had a two-cup size difference between my breasts. I was advised to get a breast form to fill out my bra and compensate for the weight disparity. The first time I went for a fitting I had a horrible experience. The dressing room was dark, dingy, and cramped, and the woman who was my fitter was so ancient and infirm that she could barely walk into this inadequate space. The lady did not take my height into consideration—I am a petite five-foot-three—nor did she understand my need to feel feminine and attractive. First she wanted to fit me with an ugly, enormous bra that extended practically from my neck to my waist. Then she brought in a huge, heavy breast form. I literally started crying and ran out without making a purchase.

After asking around during the next few days, I found someone who'd had a wonderful experience with a trained certified fitter. My friend told me that she had cried with joy when she was handed her first bra at the store because it was black lace and very sexy. With the form inside the bra she looked just as she had before her mastectomy. In fact, she felt so proud to be a woman wearing her new prosthesis that when she went home that evening she did a near-naked modeling of it for her partner.

When I went to see the same fitter, I was placed in a beautiful, well-lit, and comfortable room where I was shown a variety of lace bras and a tiny breast form that was just the right size to help fill out my smaller side. I tried on a number of bras until the fitter and I were both satisfied with the end result. It went a long way toward restoring my confidence and sense of femininity.

Not wearing a breast form or wearing one that is heavier or lighter than your existing breast can throw off your equilibrium and may result in spinal curvature, shoulder drops, muscle contractions, and issues with balance. Similarly, an improperly fitting prosthesis is uncomfortable and can contribute to these concerns.

Sandra Saffle, the National Prosthesis Coordinator for Nordstrom, suggests the following basic guidelines for a properly fitting breast form and bra:

1. Make sure the bra fits and supports you, hugging your chest wall, the underside of your arms, and your cup area. Your flesh should neither overflow from the top of the bra nor from beneath your underarms. If you have an existing breast, make sure the bra cup has the capacity to contain the full breast. Then the prosthesis form for the other side can be sized appropriately to match.

2. The bottom of the bra should be comfortably snug and anchored low on the small of the

back, rather than across the shoulder blades. The front of the bra band should fit flush against your chest wall all the way to the center tacks. There should be no gaping or bowing along the top of it.

3. Your bra straps should not cut into the tops of your shoulders since the bra should be supporting you from under your bust line, rather than pulling from the top.

4. For a bilateral fit, try a style with a fuller band on the bottom to help anchor the bra, and fuller coverage on the top edge so your breast forms won't fall away from your body when you bend forward.

Breast forms come in various shapes, sizes, and colors to accommodate different body types, breast shapes, surgeries, and personal preference. They may be manufactured from silicone, foam, or fiberfill. Generally these fit into bras that are lined with special pockets to hold them in place.

Another option is to wear a breast form that attaches directly to your body. Many women prefer the freedom of movement introduced by an attachable form, since in this case the weight of the form is on the front of the body instead of the shoulders. An added benefit is the reduced risk of triggering lymphedema symptoms from the pressure of heavy bra straps cutting into your circulation. A new technology has given breast cancer survivors a breast form that has a silicone gel strip that enables it to adhere to the chest wall on its own.

Choose the option that works best for you. Then go ahead and buy yourself a sexy bra in your favorite color. Follow your heart and enjoy being a woman.

A FINAL NOTE Please remember always to perform the Focus on Healing exercises while wearing your breast form since you want your muscles to become accustomed to its weight and shape. It is also a good idea to check your physical alignment in the mirror once a day, say every morning when you are brushing your teeth. Take a moment to notice if one of your shoulders is higher than the other. Or have a friend walk around you once in a while to give you external feedback about whether or not you are rolling your shoulders forward.

To address specific postural or balance problems that may arise while adjusting to a new prosthesis, practice the Developing Balance exercise routine (pp. 101–109).

COPING WITH
RADIATION THERAPY

*T*he worst part of radiation therapy for me was being bone tired. Because I am such a doer and go-getter, it was very hard for me to slow down, take it easy, and keep asking for help. Still, that was exactly what I needed to do most. The lesson in this was to pamper myself and to let others pamper me.

Remember that often the best gift you can give to someone who cares about you is to allow him or her to do something for you. People feel so helpless because they cannot cure you or undergo treatment for you. But they can help . . . so let them.

Now that I am fully recovered I assure you that I have been able to return the favors of my supporters many times over. My memory of how hard it was to cope has motivated me to step up to the plate for other women in the same situation and demonstrate my appreciation. The more we can take care of each other when we feel low, the more we create a better world to live in. One of the best gifts of cancer survival is connection.

Here are a few simple ideas and strategies for coping with your radiation therapy:

♦ Take an active role in planning and participating in your treatments. You are still in charge of your life. Your voice matters. No one knows what you need better than you do, so you are responsible for telling people. Participating fully means everything can go smoother and you will feel less like a victim. Ask questions!

♦ Before you start radiation therapy, write down any questions you have about what's going to happen during treatment and when your treatment is over. Give a copy to your therapist and your doctor so they can read along as you ask the questions. Do not be afraid or feel foolish about asking any question. I guarantee that you are not the first person to ask. Believe me, they have heard it all.

♦ Schedule your treatments for a time of day that suits you best. For me this was generally early in the morning, since I discovered that my treatments always seemed to catch up with me in the afternoon. I needed a couple of hours in the middle of the day to get my errands done and make phone calls before I would start feeling poorly.

♦ Line up drivers to bring you to your radiation sessions or take a taxi. You may become too fatigued to drive yourself. There is no reason ever to worry needlessly about getting home.

♦ Have someone set up a care calendar for you. Ask a well-organized friend or family member to be your care coordinator and handle the arrangements for whatever you require during this difficult period. Give a list of all your friends and any other people who told you they wanted to help to the person you have chosen. Let him or her make the calls to find you drivers, cooks, shoppers, chore people, day care, or whatever else you need. You only need to keep in contact with your care coordinator. The bonus is that you won't have to keep asking for help—someone else does that for you.

♦ Speak up about your discomfort. Tell your radiation therapist when you feel bruised or burned in the area of your treatments. Do not try to be brave or avoid making waves. Make waves.

♦ Meditate and/or visualize during your treatment sessions. I used to visualize myself in the midst of a war and the big radiation machine as my way of destroying the cancer. Because my weapon was larger and deadlier than the cancer, of course, I always won.

♦ Apply the cream the radiologist gives you in the changing room right after your treatment. This way you can start receiving its soothing benefits immediately.

♦ After treatment, go home and lie naked on your bed for half an hour with your arm over your head to expose your radiated skin to the air. This is a good time to apply more of the cream provided by the radiologist to repair your skin.

- Remember not to use baby powder or deodorant that contains aluminum.
- Rest after your treatment session. If you have the option, go home and take a nap.
- Drink a lot of water.
- At night before you to go bed, open a vitamin E capsule and squeeze the contents onto your radiated site. Vitamin E can prevent your skin from burning and help maintain its suppleness.
- Wear a 100 percent cotton T-shirt that's one size too small under your other clothes in order to protect your radiated skin from clothing friction. When your skin becomes sensitive even gentle rubbing can be terribly irritating.

- Keep laughing. Your positive attitude is an important ally right now. Watch funny movies, read uplifting books, and listen to inspiring tapes.
- Be kind to yourself.
- Let people love you.
- Keep a special calendar at home devoted to monitoring your radiation sessions. Mark off each day of your treatment with a big red "X." Premark your last radiation session with a huge, colorful sticker to celebrate the end. When I would look at my calendar, I was always reminded that my treatment would soon be over and felt encouraged to move forward to the beginning of a positive new phase of my life.

COPING WITH CHEMOTHERAPY

"I would not have chosen any other course of treatment because it seemed so clear in my case that this was the best one for me. Yet it was difficult. I have no idea how people manage to survive without a multilevel support system. I found myself coming out of the experience with newfound appreciation of life itself and all the wonderful people who loved me and supported me through it."

—Judi, fifty-one

*B*eing breast cancer survivors places us in a unique sisterhood. I have noticed that the women in my classes generally spend the break times sharing their personal stories and swapping tips. That generosity of spirit is inspiring and makes me feel proud. As survivors we have much in common and many opportunities to connect and learn from one another.

Chemotherapy generally continues over a period of six months to a year and at times can be debilitating, both physically and emotionally. Finding support from other survivors is especially important during this difficult phase of your treatment. But life goes on and your humanity is going to shine through any awkward moments.

Your chemotherapy may even surprise you with a good laugh, such as when the eleven-year-old son of an acquaintance was acting bratty. This woman had been through three treatments and still had a full head of hair. Without thinking and out of exasperation, she jokingly threatened her kid, "If you don't stop doing that, I'm going to tear my hair out." At that same moment she put her hands to her head in make-believe. Lo and behold, she came back with two big clumps of hair in her hands. She and her son were both so shocked that they started to laugh and then to cry together.

None of the tips and strategies you'll find in this section is complicated. These are just a handful of practical ideas other survivors have come up with or discovered through experience. They range from ideas for coping with your doctors and your anxiety, to how to make yourself more comfortable and handle the unpleasant side effects of treatment.

I hope these tips help make your life a little easier.

♦ Establish a good working relationship with the nursing staff in your oncologist's office. Nurses have easy access to doctors for quick input. It also helps to be able to phone them to discuss the kinds of issues that can come up. They know many ways to manage the side effects of chemotherapy, including finding the right mix of drugs and other remedies to alleviate your nausea and discomfort.

♦ Do not listen to anyone's horror stories. Go to chemotherapy with an open mind.

♦ Learn about the process of chemotherapy. Understanding can eliminate some of your fears.

♦ Ask questions about the treatment you are on and what remedies are available to prevent side effects . . . and then use them.

♦ Drink plenty of fluids. Water flushes the chemical toxins out of your body. Fruit juices can help calm your stomach.

♦ Have someone drive you to all your treatments and bring you home again. Depending on what your chemo "cocktail" is, you may be out of it. For the same reason, be careful about doing chores when you get home.

♦ During chemotherapy, many women complain of "chemo brain," or difficulty thinking. Keep a notepad and pen with you at all times. Maintain a written log of what you do and have to do and refer back to it.

♦ When you go for treatment bring something pleasant with you to do that you enjoy and that relaxes you, such as a portable CD player to play your favorite music, some knitting, or a good book to read. One woman I know used to bring a snack.

♦ Take a friend with you to your chemotherapy session. Use the time to visit and catch up. It is a good way to let close friends "experience" the chemo room and see that it's not so scary. It helps them see that you're OK while undergoing chemo and also makes the time pass a lot faster.

- Visualize healing images during your treatment sessions. Think of a golden healing fluid coming into your body that is melting away all the cancer in its path. Celebrate each chemo treatment as a positive healing experience.

- One woman I know found the word *chemo* frightening. By always referring to it as "medicine" she was able to transform her unpleasant images into healing ones.

- Keep copies of all the reports you receive and read your medical chart regularly. Ask questions about whatever you don't understand. These reports pertain to your welfare.

- Nausea and vomiting are common problems during chemotherapy. In addition to the antiemetic medication usually prescribed by cancer centers, try eating small, frequent meals. Select low-fat, bland foods and avoid those that can cause gas. Avoid lying down immediately after eating. You may also find that eating a light meal right before your treatment helps.

- Consume extra protein when bringing your blood counts back up. Eat smaller and more frequent meals, if necessary.

- Mouth sores are a common problem, so keep your mouth clean. Use a soft toothbrush and gel toothpaste and floss daily. Rinse your mouth out with club soda every two to four hours. Avoid commercial mouthwashes, smoking, alcohol, and candy and gum that contains concentrated sugars. You can also use a water-soluble cream, such as K-Y Jelly, on dry lips. Lip balms or lipsticks may be helpful, too, so long as they are water-based and do not contain alcohol or astringents.

- Another side effect of chemotherapy is constipation. Increase the fiber in your diet by eating vegetables, fruit, and whole-grain foods.

- Ask a friend who is very organized to be your care coordinator. Give this person a list of people who have offered to help you—coworkers, friends, relatives. Make a "dream" list itemizing what kinds of things you need done. Examples might be car rides, chores, shopping, day care, cooking, and companionship. Let your care coordinator contact these volunteers and then put together a calendar for the month. Everyone's name and phone number will be written down on the calendar, telling you what they are going to do for you on specific days.

- Practice your religion. Research at Duke University's Center for the Study of Religion/Spirituality and Health shows that people who pray and attend religious services rebound faster from illness and handle depression better than those who don't have as strong a sense of faith. It makes no difference what faith you practice.

- Do regular exercise during your treatment period. It can help you feel better. One survivor I know always made sure she got out to walk. Breathing fresh air and getting her blood circulating helped to combat the side effects of her chemotherapy.

- Prior to starting chemotherapy, get a wig. If you buy a wig before your hair falls out, you can match your hair color and find a style that works without feeling self-conscious about being bald. There is not always a lot of time. Your hair could fall out as early as the second session.

- Alternatively, to assume control and maintain your privacy, you may choose to shave your head before chemotherapy makes your hair fall out. Begin to wear a wig prior to your treatments and no one ever needs to know when or if you have lost your hair.

- To welcome your hair falling out and any other side effects, remind yourself that this means the chemo is working. This is a time-limited process, like a pregnancy, so imagine that you are pregnant and giving birth to your new life.

- Wear something comfortable and cheery. Taking the time to look good when you feel awful can actually make you feel better. The American Cancer Society has a national program called Look Good Feel Better that offers free makeup and makeup lessons, free consultations on wigs, and tips on how to wear a scarf around your head. Call to register: (800) ACS-2345; in Canada, (800) 914-5665.

- Make sure people understand the fatigue factor related to chemotherapy if you are working during this period. Consider cutting back your hours. It is important that you allow yourself extra down time. Rest and relaxation are essential for healing.

- Insomnia can be a problem. Stay away from caffeine. Take naps during the day. And avoid strenuous activity right before bedtime.

- Keep a journal. Writing down your emotions and clearing your thoughts can help ease any inner turmoil you may be experiencing. Journaling gives you a reference point by enabling you to identify patterns of thought, feeling, and responses to the treatment.

- Read uplifting survivor stories. Hearing what someone else has gone through can affirm your own feelings and bring you comfort.

- Find a support group or a person you can have a heart-to-heart talk with. Fellow cancer patients and survivors naturally understand what you are going through. Your hospital should have some recommendations for you, or see Finding Support (p. 257).

- Get a massage. Massage can help to release the chemical toxins from your body and also eases the aches and pains that come from lying in bed for longer amounts of time.

- Do a little "retail" therapy. You don't need to spend a lot of money or make a huge dent in your wallet; nonetheless, it can be fun to reward yourself with small gifts from time to time.

- Be positive. Have a sense of humor and keep laughing. Negative thoughts can be destructive.

MAMMOGRAPHY AND SELF-EXAMINATION AFTER BREAST CANCER DIAGNOSIS

*E*arly detection of cancer saves lives. Therefore breast cancer survivors need to get regular mammograms or ultrasounds and also perform monthly breast self-examinations. Alarmingly, I have found through casual polling at my workshops that many survivors do neither. Apparently some women avoid these evaluations out of fear or denial of what they could discover—as if the test would cause the dreaded disease. Others believe that it is impossible to have a recurrence in the chest wall on your surgical side—this is a myth. And too many women simply forget or procrastinate—yet the sooner a woman knows she has a lump, the better her prospects become for living. And if she is perfectly healthy, the test can help put her mind at ease.

Why worry needlessly? Why not be proactive and pragmatic about your health and future? Routine exams make sense and can make a difference.

I don't mean to downplay anyone's fear. I get scared, too. Fear is there from the moment I see the date on my calendar until I actually go. When my mother was alive, she and my aunt would go to their mammograms together for team support. Then they would go celebrate after they got their "all clear."

The part I hate most is when the radiologist is done and I am sitting in one of those awful gowns that sometimes close and sometimes don't. Often the radiologist comes back out and says, "Could we take some more pictures?" My mind begins to work overtime and I'm already planning for surgery and telling my family, "We have to go through this again." After the third year of extra films, I pleaded, "Just tell me if you see something!" Of course they can't do that. So now I see my doctor on the same day as the mammogram so that I don't have to go through that horrible ordeal of waiting.

MAMMOGRAPHY For the first year after surgery, your doctors will probably recommend having a mammogram every six months, then going back on a regular annual schedule. The mammogram is the most popular method of breast screening.

Ultrasound is sometimes used as a follow-up to mammography when breast tissue is denser and more nodular than average—as is often the case with younger women—or when something suspicious emerges on an initial mammogram.

New technologies are being researched in order to detect cancer at an earlier (smaller) stage of development. Most are not yet available.

Women who have had reconstructive surgery with a saline implant cannot be screened by mammography or ultrasound on that side. In this case, you must rely on breast self-examination in the area around your implant.

SELF-EXAMINATION Women find most breast lumps, and most turn out not to be cancerous. A monthly self-examination gives you the opportunity to learn what your normal breast tissue and surgical site feel like and thus increases your ability to notice changes. Self-exams are incredibly easy and should take only a few minutes.

Some women do not believe it is possible to have a lump when breast tissue has been completely removed. Please don't make this mistake. Thankfully my close friend Becky caught a new lump on her surgical side five years after her mastectomy by taking the time to do a breast exam. Because she found the cancer early, she is doing well today.

The best time to do a self-exam is a few days (three to five) after your period, since women's breasts are typically less swollen and lumpy then. If you have stopped menstruating, or your period sometimes skips a month, you should pick a day for your exam. Just make sure it is the same day every month. I use my birth date because it is an easy number to remember. You could also choose the first or the fifteenth of the month.

You should examine your breasts and/or chest wall, including the lymph node area. At the beginning, when you are learning, you may want to practice with your doctor and have him or her help you figure out what you are feeling. That way it will be easier to distinguish the normal feeling of your scar tissue and what else is present at your surgical site. Your doctor should do a breast examination during your regular office visits, too.

The American Cancer Society recommends the following guidelines for breast self-examination. If you find any changes during your monthly exam, see your doctor right away. Trust your instincts—no one knows your body as well as you—and don't be afraid to ask questions.

1. Lie down and place a pillow under your right shoulder. Put the right arm behind your head. This elevates and exposes your right breast and underarm.

2. Use the pads of the three middle fingers on your left hand to feel for lumps and thickening in your right breast.

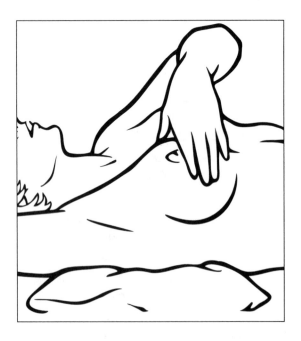

3. Press firmly enough to know how your breast feels. Your goal is to learn what's normal. A firm ridge in the lower curve of each breast is normal, for example. If you have had radiation therapy, you might feel some lumpiness under your surgical scar or some firmness or puckering.

4. Move around the breast in one of three set patterns: circles, vertical lines, or a wedge. Do the exam the same way every time. Cover the entire breast area and armpit.

   ◆ To make circles, start on the outside of the breast and feel around it in ever-narrowing circles until you reach the nipple.
   ◆ To make vertical lines, start on one side of the breast and feel down it in a line and then move across it slightly and feel up it. Go up and down until you have covered the entire breast territory.
   ◆ To follow a wedge, start on the outside of the breast and feel inward along a line that ends at the nipple. Then keep moving your starting point around your breast as though it were the face of a clock. Begin at one o'clock, then two o'clock, and so on.

5. Now examine your left breast in the same way using your right finger pads.

6. Repeat the self-examination of both breasts while standing with your arm behind your head. Being upright makes it easier to check the upper and lower parts of your breasts near your armpit. Do this part of your exam while you are in the shower and slippery with water

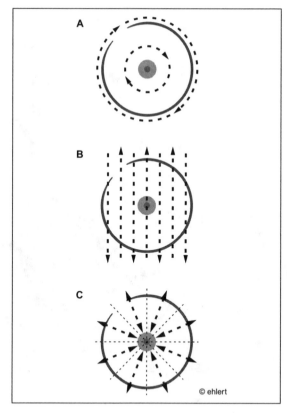

© ehlert

and soap lather. Another option is to do it while standing in front of a mirror.

7. Finally, check both breasts in the mirror for any visual signs of dimpling in the skin, changes in the nipple, redness, or swelling.

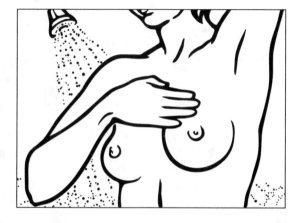

Changes to look for:

◆ Anything different from what is normal for your breasts.

◆ Lumps could feel hard, round, elongated, or like a "thickening."

◆ Skin discoloration, dimpling, itching, rashes, an orange peel appearance, or veins that suddenly become prominent.

◆ A sore that won't heal or swelling.

◆ An inverted nipple or nipple discharge.

BREAST MAPPING Kim Schaaf, a breast educator and consultant with several hospitals in the Seattle, Washington, area, introduced me to breast mapping. The idea is to make notes each month about what you find during your routine self-examination. It makes it a lot easier to remember the details and, if necessary, to share them with your doctor.

Ask your doctor to help you establish a baseline by giving you a breast examination. Have your doctor mark down on the diagram (p. 256) any normal lumps he or she finds. From then on you can compare and mark down what you notice during your monthly self-exams, particularly anything that you are not sure about. For your monthly notes, describe what you feel in your own words so that it makes sense to you when you read it a month later. Each month, refer back to what your doctor drew and you wrote, and then add any new findings.

Should you happen to find a lump that is not a part of your baseline, consult your doctor about it right away. Trust your instincts.

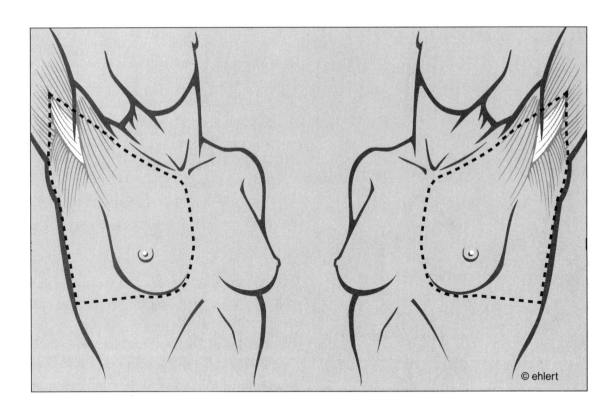

January: _____

February: _____

March: _____

April: _____

May: _____

June: _____

July: _____

August: _____

September: _____

October: _____

November: _____

December: _____

FINDING SUPPORT

*E*veryone needs emotional support. Support is not the same as help with cooking, shopping, child care, and other daily tasks, although these are important. Help may be essential to you when you are in treatment and recovery—after all, you are not Superwoman—but it is not the only thing you need. You also need love and affection, someone to listen and acknowledge your feelings, and someone to encourage you and be proud of your efforts. No one is an island. Cancer is a challenging life experience, one that brings up fear, grief, and a sense of loss of control. Support can help you handle these stresses.

When you were first diagnosed, you probably needed help making choices about your treatment options. That could have come from a spouse, a grown child, a sister, or a friend. You may have wanted that someone to sit beside you while you spoke to your doctors, perhaps taking notes to help you remember and evaluate the avalanche of information that was rapidly pouring over you. Now, since you are reading this book, I am assuming that you are either in radiation or chemotherapy, or you have completed your treatment. You may be a long-term survivor. Depending on which phase you are in, the support and help you need could vary.

FAMILY AND FRIENDS Women who are still in treatment are going through a rigorous process. It demands you call upon all your personal resources. There will be good days and bad days. Your emotions may overwhelm you. It is important that you communicate your feelings honestly and openly to your family and friends. Let them know how you are right now, so they don't have to guess. Share when you need a hug, a shoulder to lean on, an ear to listen, or a period of solitude.

For me, my husband was my rock, my support, and my source of affection. He told me that he did not marry me for the outer shell. All that mattered to him was that my inside was still the same. He was there for me at every turn in the road. He was my nurse when they sent me home from the hospital, my sounding board when I needed someone to hear me, and he understood my deepest fears. Another woman I know came home from the hospital to an empty house. Her husband had left a note apologizing for leaving her, saying he couldn't cope. Some of us are lucky to have the support of a good man or a good woman. Others of us must find other sources of support.

Keep in mind that your family and friends are going through a whole series of emotional responses as well. Sometimes our partners, other caregivers, and children need help coming to terms with their own feelings about our cancer.

Sadly, not everyone is prepared or able to offer support. But those who are willing and able to be with us during the experience are like angels.

My friend Judi is a bus driver who had a mastectomy at age fifty-two. Her job demanded that she be able to turn a huge wheel—and rapidly at times—a movement that calls upon the muscles in the front and sides of the body. It took Judi longer than average to get back her range of motion because of complications from her surgery. She had to take several months off and when she resumed working could only work part-time for another six months.

Judi's story has a happy ending. Many people on her job donated some of their paid leave time to her, including sick days and vacation days, so that she wouldn't have to worry about finances during her recovery. Thoughtful, caring coworkers sent cards, gifts, prayers, and good wishes. She was extremely fortunate that her employers and her coworkers took such good care of her and that she had a job to go back to when she recovered. That community of support made a huge difference.

Women who have completed treatment generally need some time to integrate the experience into their lives. You have moved from decision-making, through treatment, and now to survival. Your doctors, nurses, and other professional supporters have faded into the background, and as a result you may feel surprisingly isolated. There may be fears of recurrence. Again, your loved ones can be a tremendous source of comfort. A supportive spouse or friend can be a valuable ally in everything you do.

You may also be struggling with meaning. Questions may come up about your identity and what you want out of life. Lots of survivors make changes and come to see cancer as a pivotal event. Some switch careers, others end marriages. It can be a wakeup call that brings you an opportunity to live a more positive and meaningful future.

So where can you and your family get appropriate support? Knowing where to turn is not always easy. But ignoring your feelings won't make them go away. Too many survivors practice denial, hiding their pain behind a happy face. Sometimes it is important to take the gamble and reach out and say, "This is what's bothering me and I need some help with it."

If you have been comparing yourself to someone who you think is wonderful and brave and seems to have it all under control, I'll let you in on a little secret. She has probably had help along the way—and there's nothing wrong with that!

SUPPORT GROUPS Finding a support group that fits you is like shopping for a new outfit. What works for some women does not work for others. I visited several support groups during my treatment and never did seem to locate the right one. Yet my good friend Judi loves her support group and would not miss a weekly meeting. She has been going for almost two years now. Hers is an educational group sponsored by the hospital where she had surgery. The group has speakers and presenters come in and talk to them about various subjects. Their facilitator is a vibrant, upbeat, and enthusiastic woman who leads the group to success.

Some support groups are geared toward younger women, some toward older women. Some take the form of social gatherings and are forums of discussion. Others deal with their members' issues of the moment. My advice is to shop around. Visit a few groups and then choose. Your hospital, doctors, and the local American Cancer Society office can provide you with lists of groups in your area.

There are also support groups available for the spouses and children of women with breast cancer. Ask the same sources for advice on how to locate these.

Please do not be deterred from going to support groups or attending exercise programs because you are fifteen years down the road from your original surgery. Your issues may persist and you may still have questions. Just because you are not a "new" survivor doesn't mean you still won't have cancer issues, old and new.

COUNSELORS If a support group is not your cup of tea, you can also meet privately with the social worker in your hospital's oncology unit to discuss your feelings and needs. They are a wonderful resource, so use them. Oftentimes their services are free to patients.

A good psychologist can also provide you with a safe place to speak out and address feelings you might not feel comfortable discussing "in a crowd." I went to see a wonderful therapist for one-on-one counseling; she helped me confront my fears of death and dying. In her office I was able to cry and not hold anything back. It was just what I needed to come to terms with my fears and move on.

Your doctor or the local American Cancer Society office should be able to provide you with references to good therapists. Ask your friends if they know one. It is important that you feel comfortable talking to the therapist you select.

HOT LINES There are many breast cancer support phone lines, where you can get answers to questions from other survivors. A survivor can often tell you things your doctor might not even know. When I was in radiation I had problems with nerves that had been cut during surgery that gave me shooting pain for weeks. It was agonizing and perplexing at first. Then I called a hot line number and spoke to a woman who was a wonderful listener and had gone through a similar experience. She encouraged me to hang in and not give up hope and made a good suggestion to ease my discomfort. Sure enough, the nerve pain was temporary. That support got me through a rough spot.

Here are the numbers of a few toll-free hot lines you may contact (also see Resources):

◆ (800) 4CANCER
◆ American Cancer Society: (800) ACS-2345
◆ Y-ME: (800) 221-2141; and in Spanish: (800) 986-9505
◆ The Wellness Community: (888) 783-WELL

For your informational needs, many hospitals have cancer wellness centers staffed with volunteers trained to answer your questions. These include libraries full of videotapes and books on topics of interest.

CHURCHES, SYNAGOGUES, AND MOSQUES

Most religious institutions today have counselors on staff trained to listen and offer assistance. Such a counselor could be a priest, pastor, rabbi, or layperson. The spiritual leader of your personal house of worship will likely counsel you for free. Some other religious service organizations, such as Catholic Family Services and Jewish Family Services, offer counseling on a sliding scale fee. So please do not feel that because funds are tight there is no place for you to go.

Contact your church, synagogue, or mosque and ask for a referral. Your hospital social worker can also help direct you to an appropriate counseling service. Go to them, get the help you need, and do not feel bad about asking.

Even if you don't desire one-on-one counseling, going to a regular weekly worship service has proven healthful. The connection to community and the connection to God through prayer are powerful.

ACTIVITIES

There are organizations across the United States and Canada that provide group activities for cancer survivors. In Seattle, where I live, I know offhand about groups where you can enjoy art, music, writing, gentle yoga, walking, and biking. During my radiation therapy I joined a knitting group. The lessons and materials were free and so was the companionship of the other survivors. They helped me because I always felt I had a place to turn. Whatever your favorite hobby is, there is probably a group that pursues it. These groups give you the opportunity to do what makes you happy in the company of people who are in a similar position. For the most part these activities are free.

A physician-approved exercise class can be another key to emotional freedom. My personal breast cancer experience heightened my awareness of how important the Focus on Healing program could be to survivors in every stage of recovery. Choose a program that is gentle and kind to your body and soul, rather than overly strenuous. When you get your endorphins going, you should feel lighter, freer, and laugh more. While you are having fun, you are doing something special for yourself inside and out.

Another option is to join a meditation group. Through meditation you can learn more about who you are inside and practice self-acceptance in the presence of gentle, loving company. Remember, you have a chance to be good to yourself . . . and it can be a wonderful adventure.

A FINAL NOTE

*I*t is my honor to share the Focus on Healing program with you. I am excited that you have taken this important step to care for your body, your mind, and your spirit. You and I have something in common. We've struggled and fought with cancer and we've survived. Now it's our time to thrive. We do this by living our lives to the fullest; reaching out every day to friends, family, and other survivors; being active; and doing what we need to do to heal physically and emotionally. Progress doesn't happen overnight, but in time and with persistence we go on and get better, stronger, and happier.

Music and dance offer an experience of freedom, grace, and happiness. I believe that when we move we feel most alive, our hearts soar, and we reclaim ourselves. If I were with you right now, I would give you a big hug and a kiss and a pat on the back. I'd tell you the same thing I tell all my students at the end of class:

You're strong.

You're beautiful.

You're feminine.

You're courageous.

You're more than a survivor—you are a thriver!

So please remember to laugh and do something wonderful every day. And save the next dance for me!

RESOURCES

FOR EXERCISE PROGRAMS AND SPORTING ACTIVITIES

To inquire about the location of a Focus on Healing class in your community in the United States, and/or receive training and certification as a program instructor, or to order a *Rhythmic Accompaniments to Focus on Healing Through Movement and Dance* class CD, please contact:

Focus on Healing Through Movement and
    Dance for the Breast Cancer Survivor
14418 47th Place West
Lynnwood, WA 98037
Telephone: (877) 365-6014 (toll free)
Website: www.focusonhealing.net

In Canada, to find a Focus on Healing class contact:

Complementary Cancer Choices
359 Scenic Acres Drive NW
Calgary, AB T3L 1T6
Telephone: (877) 773-2825 (toll free) or (403)
    241-2825
Website: www.money4cancer.com

This organization also provides education on complementary cancer therapies and financial assistance to Canadian women to pay for therapies not covered by health plans.

The Focus on Healing videotape is available through:

Enhancement, Inc.
Telephone: (888) 584-9633 (toll free)
Website: www.enhancementinc.com

The American College of Sports Medicine can refer you to a registered clinical exercise physiologist specializing in the needs of oncology patients. You can also ask your oncologist for a similar referral. These are allied health professionals who work with clients and patients who have diseases and conditions where exercise is proven to be beneficial, including cancer. Contact:

American College of Sports Medicine
Telephone: (317) 637-9200
Website: www.acsm.org

Cancer Lifeline offers exercise programs, such as yoga, tai chi, and dance therapy, and emotional support groups for breast cancer survivors. Contact:

Cancer Lifeline
Telephone: 800-255-5500 (national toll free)
    or (206) 297-2500 (Washington State toll
    free)
Website: www.cancerlifeline.com

Team Survivor is an organization whose mission is to maximize the participation of women cancer survivors in physical activity and fitness programs. Their activities are open to women of all ages and fitness levels and in all stages of treatment and recovery. To find a local chapter it is easiest to visit the website; however, you may also telephone to be directed to an appropriate contact in your area.

Team Survivor
Telephone: (310) 829-7849
Website: www.teamsurvivor.org
Team Survivor Seattle
Telephone: (206) 732-8450

The Encore Plus program of the YWCA of the United States offers exercise programs, such as swimming, watersize, yoga, dance therapy, and tai chi, and other services for breast cancer survivors. Check your phone book to find a local YWCA, or contact:

YWCA
624 9th Street NW, 3rd Floor
Washington, DC 20001-5303
Telephone: (900) 95-EPLUS (toll free)
Website: www.ywca.org

The models in this book are wearing sportswear generously donated by the following two suppliers. For more information and to place an order, contact:

Cobblestones Active Wear
Telephone: (800) 592-7195 (toll free)
Website: www.cobblestones.com

Jacques Moret Sportswear
Telephone: (800) 441-1999 (toll free)
Website: www.moret.com

FOR SUPPORT

The American Cancer Society offers a twenty-four-hour hot line and referrals for all types of issues and needs, free literature relating to breast cancer and treatment, and advice on where to locate pertinent research. Their Reach to Recovery program is run by a group of breast cancer survivors who volunteer time to visit newly diagnosed women and recent surgical survivors to help guide them to the resources they need (see also Look Good Feel Better, p. 264).
Your local ACS chapter can put you in touch. Contact:

American Cancer Society
1599 Clifton Road NE
Atlanta, GA 30329
Telephone: (800) ACS-2345 (toll free)
Website: www.cancer.org

The sister organization of the American Cancer Society is the Canadian Cancer Society. They offer similar services. Contact:

Canadian Cancer Society, National Office
10 Alcorn Avenue, Suite 200
Toronto, Ontario M4V 3B1
Telephone: (416) 961-7223
Website: www.cancer.ca

Cancer Care maintains an extensive list of community-based resources in your area. For more information, contact:

Cancer Care
Telephone: (800) 813-HOPE (toll free)
Website: www.cancercare.org

Cancer Connection offers phone links to other breast cancer survivors who have similar diagnoses. Contact:

Cancer Connection
Telephone (800) 263-6750 (toll free)

In Canada, Cancer Information Services provides information on cancer and cancer resources. Contact:

Cancer Information Services
328 Mountain Park Avenue, 3rd floor
Hamilton, Ontario L8V 4X2
Telephone: (888) 939-3333 (toll free, bilingual)
    or (905) 387-1153

The Celebrating Life Foundation is a national organization that promotes breast cancer awareness among African-American women and women of color. They offer educational material, workshops, local support groups, and numerous other resources. Contact:

Celebrating Life Foundation
PO Box 224076
Dallas, TX 75222
Telephone: (800) 207-0992 (toll free)
Website: www.celebratinglife.org

Gilda's Club (named for Gilda Radner) is a national support community for men, women, and children living with cancer, and their families and friends. All services are free. Contact Gilda's Club Seattle for a location and state near you.

Gilda's Club Seattle
info@gildasclubseattle.org
Telephone: (206) 709-1400

The Komen Foundation has a mission to eradicate breast cancer as a life-threatening disease by advancing research, education, screenings, and treatment. The IM-AWARE telephone hot line is a wonderful all-around resource. Contact:

Susan G. Komen Breast Cancer Foundation
5005 L.B.J. Freeway, Suite 370
Dallas, TX 75244
Telephone: (800) IM-AWARE (toll free) or
    (972) 855-1600
Website: www.komen.org

Living Beyond Breast Cancer promotes the health of women affected by breast cancer through workshops, newsletters, conferences, and a telephone help line. Contact:

Living Beyond Breast Cancer
10 East Athens Avenue, Suite 204
Ardmore, PA 19003
Telephone: (610) 645-4567

In Canada, Living Well with Cancer is a partnership of those living with cancer and health care professionals. They provide fact sheets. Contact:

Living Well with Cancer
Telephone: (877) 909-5992 (toll free)

Look Good Feel Better is a program offered in the United States by the American Cancer Society and in Canada. They give free workshops on how to camouflage the appearance-related side effects of cancer using makeup, wigs, and scarves. Talented cosmeticians volunteer their time to this program, and the makeup products they give away can be worth as much as $300. Two years after treatment they welcomed me with open arms. I had fun and left feeling beautiful. Contact:

American Cancer Society
Telephone: (800) ACS-2345 (toll free)
Canada Look Good Feel Better
Telephone: (800) 914-5665 (toll free)

The Mautner Project is the only national organization dedicated to lesbians with cancer, their partners, and caregivers. They provide direct services and education, and pursue advocacy. Contact:

Mautner Project for Lesbians with Cancer
1707 L Street NW, Suite 500
Washington DC 20036
Telephone: (202) 323-5536
Website: www.mautnerproject.org

NABCO is the leading nonprofit information and education resource on breast cancer with a network of over four hundred member organizations across the United States. They provide information to medical professionals and their organizations and to patients and their families. Contact:

National Alliance of Breast Cancer
    Organizations
9 East 37th Street, 10th Floor
New York, NY 10016
Telephone: (888) 80-NABCO (toll free)
Website: www.nabco.org

NBCC is a grassroots advocacy organization dedicated to fighting breast cancer. They offer guidance on finding quality cancer care throughout the United States.

National Breast Cancer Coalition
1707 L Street NW, Suite 1060
Washington DC 20036
Telephone: (202) 296-7477
Website: www.natlbcc.org

Reach to Recovery is a program offered in the United States by the American Cancer Society and in Canada. Volunteers make visits to newly diagnosed women and recent surgical survivors. Contact:

American Cancer Society
Telephone: (800) ACS-2345 (toll free)
Reach to Recovery Canada
Telephone: (888) 939-3333 (toll free)

Sisters of Hope is a support group for African-American women with breast cancer and their families. Telephone the Washington State chapter to receive a contact number in your own area.

Sisters of Hope
c/o Betty Mewborn
2531 South J Street
Tacoma, WA 98405
Telephone: (253) 572-2683
E-mail: sistersofhope@hotmail.com

The mission of the Wellness Community is to help people with cancer and their families enhance their health and well-being by providing a professional program of emotional support, education, and hope. Contact:

The Wellness Community
35 East 7th Street, Suite 412
Cincinnati, OH 45202
Telephone: (888) 783-WELL (toll free)
Website: www.wellness-community.org

The mission of Y-ME is to decrease the impact of breast cancer, create and increase breast cancer awareness, and to ensure, through information, empowerment, and peer support, that no one faces breast cancer alone. Contact:

Y-ME National Breast Cancer Organization
212 West Van Buren Street
Chicago, IL 60607

Telephone: (800) 221-2141; (toll free) Spanish language: (800) 986-9505 (toll free)
Website: www.y-me.org

FOR LYMPHEDEMA

National Lymphedema Network can put you in touch with a lymphedema therapist, doctors, support groups, and detailed information. If you are currently showing symptoms or are considered at-risk for lymphedema, please contact:

National Lymphedema Network
1611 Telegraph Avenue, Suite 1111
Oakland, CA 94612-2138
Telephone: (800) 541-3259 (toll free)
Website: www.lymphnet.org

FOR FREE OR LOW-COST MAMMOGRAPHY

The American Cancer Society may be able to direct you to a resource in your community. Call (800) ACS-2345. You could also speak to the social work department in your hospital, your doctor, or a local clinic to see if they know of inexpensive mammography options. It may take some research to locate them.

AICF runs the Free Mobile Mammography Program to serve underprivileged New York–area women with no-cost screenings. For more information, please contact:

American-Italian Cancer Foundation
112 East 71st Street, 2B
New York, NY 10021
Telephone: (212) 628-9090
Website: aicfonline.org

SHARE, in addition to providing support groups and Focus on Healing exercise programs in all five boroughs of New York City, this organization can refer women over fifty, as well as women over forty who have no health insurance, for free mammograms through their Breast Health Partnerships program.

SHARE
1501 Broadway, Suite 1720
New York, NY 10036
Telephone: (212) 719-0364
Website: www.sharecancersupport.org

FOR PROSTHETIC BREASTS

Amoena is a division of Coloplast, Inc. As manufacturers of prosthetic breasts, they can direct you to retail sources and a certified fitter in your area. For assistance, contact:

Amoena
Telephone: (800) 788-0293 (toll free)
Website: www.thebreastcaresite.com

Nordstrom is a national department store that has made an effort to provide trained and certified prosthetic fitters across the United States. When you call them ask to be referred to the Prosthesis Coordinator.

Nordstrom
Telephone: (800) 804-1502 (toll free)
Website: www.nordstrom.com

Women without insurance should call their local American Cancer Society or Canadian Cancer Society offices for assistance in purchasing a breast form. Check your local phone book to find the nearest chapter.

FOR NUTRITION AND WEIGHT LOSS

The oncology social worker in your hospital can give you a referral to a nutritionist in your area. Most hospitals also have experienced nutritionists on staff.

The American Dietetic Association can give you a referral to a qualified dietitian in your area specializing in oncology. They have seventy thousand members nationwide. Contact:

American Dietetic Association
Telephone: (800) 366-1655 (toll free)
Website: www.eatright.org

RECOMMENDED READING

After Cancer: A Guide to Your New Life by Wendy Schlessel Harpham, M.D. HarperPerennial, 1995.

Be a Survivor: Your Guide to Breast Cancer Treatment, edition II by Vladimir Lange, M.D., Lange Productions, 2002.

Before the Change: Taking Charge of Your Perimenopause by Ann Louise Gittleman. HarperSanFrancisco, 1999.

Bosom Buddies: Lessons and Laughter on Breast Health and Cancer by Rosie O'Donnell and Deborah Axelrod, M.D., F.A.C.S. with Tracy Chutorian. Warner Books, 1999.

Breast Cancer in the Family? A Guide When a Woman You Love Is Diagnosed with Breast Cancer by Leah de Roulet, M.S.W. An e-book available on-line from www.mightywords.com, 2001.

Breast Fitness: An Optimal Exercise and Health Plan for Reducing Your Risk of Breast Cancer by Anne McTiernan, M.D., Ph.D.; Julie Gralow, M.D.; and Lisa Talbott. St. Martin's Press, 2000.

The Cancer Survival Cookbook: 200 Quick and Easy Recipes with Helpful Eating Hints by Donna L. Wiehofen, R.D., M.S., with Christina Marino, M.D., M.P.H. John Wiley & Sons, 1997.

Coping with Lymphedema by Joan Swirsky, R.N., and Diane Sackett Nannery. Avery Penguin Putnam, 1998.

Dr. Susan Love's Breast Book by Susan Love, M.D. Perseus Book Group, 2000.

Dr. Susan Love's Hormone Book: Making Informed Choices about Menopause by Susan Love, M.D. Random House, 1998.

Just Get Me Through This! The Practical Guide to Breast Cancer by Deborah A. Cohen. Kensington, 2000.

Living Beyond Breast Cancer: A Survivor's Guide for when Treatment Ends and the Rest of Your Life Begins by Marisa C. Weiss, M.D., and Ellen Weiss. Times Books, 1998.

Love, Medicine, and Miracles: Lessons Learned about Self-Healing from a Surgeon's Experience with Exceptional Patients by Bernie Siegel, M.D. HarperPerennial, 1990.

My Mother's Breast: Daughters Face Their Mother's Cancer by Laurie Tarkan. Taylor, 1999.

Rituals for Women Coping with Breast Cancer by Rosalie Muschal-Reinhardt, Barbara S. Mitrano, Mary Rose McCarthy, and Jeanne Brinkman Grinnan. Prism Collective, 2000.

What to Eat Now: The Cancer Lifeline Cookbook by Rachel Keim with Ginny Smith. Sasquatch Books, 1996.

When a Parent Has Cancer: A Guide to Caring for Your Children by Wendy Schlessel Harpham. HarperCollins, 1997.

ACKNOWLEDGMENTS

I am first and foremost grateful to my husband, Jeff Davis, for encouraging me to follow my dreams and sharing me with so many others. Thank you. I love you very much. Thanks also to my sons, Adam Gloss and Randy Gloss, who have always believed in me, loved me, and let me be myself; my grandchildren, Jeremy and Jacob; my daughters-in-law, Tobey and Annissa, who share my passion; and Cathy and Iris Lebed. I am also grateful to Mikki Williams, my friend, who taught me always to ask (and I did!); Aunt Eilene, who gave me my survivor skills and taught me how to give myself to others; and Monroe and Fanette, for giving me my wheels for my covered wagon. A special thanks to Becky Robar, for being my support person through my journey as a survivor. To my friends and family, I love you all for helping me reach for the stars.

My brothers, Dr. Marc Lebed and Dr. Joel Lebed, deserve special mention for cocreating the Focus on Healing program. Marc remains the medical adviser and director of the program, which has changed so many lives, and he dedicates much of his time to do that. I love you both.

Thank you, Stephanie Gunning. You are a writer extraordinaire, my friend, and the guiding light of all these wonderful pages. Ling Lucas and Janis Donnaud, my agents, I am grateful for your belief in Focus on Healing and your passion to reach out to survivors. My appreciation goes to Nicole Brodeur, columnist, writer, and my friend; without your original story in *People* magazine there would be no book. Photographer Susan Picatti of Susan Picatti Designs, my friend, your talents have vastly enriched this book. Illustrator Dave Elhart, you have hands of gold. Barbara Cummings-Versaevel, my friend, thanks for letting me reprint your beautiful poem of welcome.

All the models for the book are breast cancer thrivers. A special thanks to Betty Mewborn, Terri Hewey, Barbara Cereghino, Debbie Makin, Vickie Rud, Jeanne Wells, Mary Giordano, Julie Kawaski, and Barbara Lee. I am deeply touched by your beauty and for giving your time to bring the Focus on Healing program to others. Many thanks also to Mark Kane of Body Balancing. Laksmi Sam, Rick Toth, Andrea Bolen, Sarah Haibeck, and Cari Lester—thank you for your time and talent in bringing out the natural radiance of these wonderful women. I would like to acknowledge Jacques Moret Sportswear and Cobblestones Active Wear for donating exercise outfits to this project.

A huge thank-you to the many survivors who have shared the personal stories, quotes, and tips that appear in this book so others could benefit from them, including Mary Paul, Diane Rosillini, Antoinette "Twin" Forbes, Phyliss

Carlson, Kathy Marshall, Patricia Piper, Karen Veasey, Janet Cross, Mary Giordano, Terri Hewey, Barbara Lee, Dana Sigley, Susan Eby, Karen Van Kirk, Linda Trenholm, Delia Mooney, Geri Robnett, Betty Mewborn, Beth Spector, and Judi Fisher.

I would like to thank my editor at Broadway Books, Ann Campbell, whose patience and knowledge led me through the unknown without fear, as well as her assistant Jenny Cookson. Thanks also to Erin Curtin, Umi Kenyon, Lisa Sloane, Jane Herman, and Lesley Krauss.

There are many individuals who gave me encouragement and advice in preparing this book and helping me deliver Focus on Healing to the world. They are experts in their fields and any errors of fact in this book are mine and not theirs. I would like to honor Jane M. Kepics, P.T., and Margaret Kleinfeld, P.T., who helped me move the program forward in the clinical world; Susan Watters, O.T.; Suzanne Dixon, epidemiologist and nutritionist; Dr. Robert Sommers; Albert Einstein Medical Center; Dr. James Blitz; Dr. Lisa Sowder; Dr. Rick Clarfeld; Shiri Rosenstein, P.T.; Deb Schiro; Lisa Talbott; Cheri Doll, P.T.; Martha Clay, A.R.N.P.; Leah DeRoulet, M.S.W.; Saskia Thiadens, R.N.; Rebecca Cook; Sandra Saffle; Michelle Correll; Kim Schaaf; Shaun Hildner, my webmaster; Swedish Medical Center in Seattle, Washington; Jody Olsen; Shoosh Crotzer; Shauna Shapiro; Emma Leybin; Sara Whitcomb; and Rita Egizii, my Canadian friend. I am indebted to every one of the enormously dedicated Focus on Healing instructors around the world, who are bringing this program to so many survivors.

To all the courageous breast cancer survivors who voiced the need for this program, I thank you for enriching my life.

INDEX

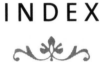